Injuries
in Outdoor
Recreation

Books by Gary N. Guten, MD

Experimental Degenerative Arthritis

How to Run Al's Run

Play Healthy, Stay Healthy

Running Injuries

Exercise, Nutrition, and Cancer

Golf Injuries: Clinics in Sports Medicine

Injuries in Outdoor Recreation

Understanding, Prevention, and Treatment

GARY N. GUTEN, MD

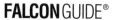

GUILFORD, CONNECTICUT
HELENA, MONTANA
AN IMPRINT OF THE GLOBE PEQUOT PRESS

Exercise directions in Part IV copyright © 2005 Covenant Healthcare System, Inc., www.covhealth.org.

Text design by Linda R. Loiewski
Illustrations on pp. 181, 182, 192, 212, and 213 by Diane Blasius

Library of Congress Cataloguing-in-Publication Data
Guten, Gary N., 1939–
    Injuries in outdoor recreation: understanding, prevention, and treatment/
Gary N. Guten.
        p. cm.
    Includes index.
    ISBN 0-7627-3676-3
        1. Outdoor medical emergencies. I. Title.
    RC88.9.O95G88 2005
    616.02'52—dc22

                                                                    20055046073

Manufactured in the United States of America
First Edition/First Printing

The author and publisher have made every effort to ensure the accuracy of the information in this book at press time. However, they cannot accept any responsibility for any loss, injury, or inconvenience resulting from the use of information contained in this guide. Readers are encouraged to seek medical help whenever possible. This book is no substitute for a physician's advice.

To my children and grandchildren:
Always listen to your body.

contents

Acknowledgments xi

Preface xiii

Part I: Listen to Your Body 1
  Why Listen to Your Body? 1
  How to Listen to Your Body 4
  Whom to Listen To 6

Part II: How to Treat an Injury 13
  What Causes Injuries? 14
  Types of Injuries 15
  Stop, Yield, Go: Learning to Listen to Your Body 17
  The 6-Point Condition Summary 17
  The 10-Point Treatment Plan 21
  Summary 39

Part III: 40 Specific Outdoor Recreational Injuries
and Treatments 43
  1. Neck—Herniated disk 47
  2. Chest—Fracture of the vertebra and rib 51
  3. Back—Herniated or slipped disk 54
  4. Back—Muscle tear 58
  5. Shoulder—Acromioclavicular joint (AC) separation 61
  6. Shoulder—Anterior dislocation 65
  7. Shoulder—Rotator cuff tendinitis and tear 69

8. Shoulder—Rupture of biceps tendon 73

9. Shoulder—Subacromial bursitis.. 76

10. Elbow—Lateral epicondylitis (tennis elbow)............................. 79

11. Elbow—Medial epicondylitis (baseball elbow) 82

12. Elbow—Ulnar nerve entrapment 85

13. Wrist—Carpal tunnel.. 88

14. Wrist—Scaphoid bone fracture (navicular bone) 91

15. Wrist—Ulnar neuritis (biker's wrist) 94

16. Finger—Extensor tendon tear (baseball finger)....................... 97

17. Finger—Ruptured ulnar collateral ligament (skier's thumb) ... 100

18. Hip—Tear of adductor muscles (inner thigh)......................... 103

19. Hip—Stress fracture of the neck of the femur 107

20. Hip—Trochanteric bursitis 111

21. Thigh—Myositis ossificans, heterotopic bone formation 114

22. Thigh—Quadriceps muscle tear... 117

23. Thigh—Hamstring muscle tear... 120

24. Knee—Anterior cruciate ligament (ACL) tear 123

25. Knee—Chondromalacia patella.. 127

26. Knee—Iliotibial band syndrome 131

27. Knee—Osgood-Schlatter disease... 134

28. Knee—Osteoarthritis.. 137

29. Knee—Kneecap (patella) dislocation 141

30. Knee—Patellar tendinitis (jumper's knee).............................. 145

31. Knee—Torn meniscus 148

32. Shin—Shin splints 151

33. Shin—Tibia or fibula stress fracture 154

34. Calf—Rupture of the gastrocnemius muscle 157

35. Ankle—Achilles tendinitis 161

36. Ankle—Torn Achilles tendon 164

37. Ankle—Lateral ligament sprain 167

38. Foot—Metatarsal stress fracture 170

39. Foot—Morton's neuroma.. 173

40. Foot—Plantar fasciitis (heel pain) 176

Part IV: Rehabilitation Exercise Programs 179

by Erin Doxtator, MPT, LAT

Upper Extremity Stretching Program 181

Lower Extremity Stretching Program 182

Back Strengthening Program 184

Beginning Shoulder Program 187

Rotator Cuff Program 190

Shoulder Acromioclavicular Program 194

Shoulder Dislocation Program 197

Lateral Epicondylitis Program—Beginning 200

Lateral Epicondylitis Program—Advanced 202

Patellar Program 204

Meniscus Program 206

Anterior Cruciate Ligament (ACL) Program 208

Ankle Program 210

Part V: Prevention of Outdoor Recreational Injuries 215

Healthy Eating for Outdoor Recreation
by Laurie Meyer, MS, RD, CD 216

Use of Poles for Fitness Walking, Hiking/Trekking,
Sports Training, and Rehabilitation
by Tom Rutlin 239

Prevention of Climbing Injuries in Hiking,
Rock Climbing, and Mountaineering
by John Loleit 253

Part VI: Orthopedic Surgery and Podiatry Management of Outdoor Recreational Injuries 261

Neck and Back Surgery for Injuries in Outdoor Recreation
by David L. Coran, MD 262

Treatment of Hand and Arm Injuries
by John A. Schneider, MD 266

Knee Pain in Recreational Biking and Running
by Harvey S. Kohn, MD 273

Twisting Injuries of the Knee in Outdoor Recreation
by Donald J. Zoltan, MD 278

Pediatric Outdoor Recreational Injuries
by Brian E. Black, MD 282

Foot Injuries in Outdoor Recreation
by Thomas A. Pietrocarlo, DPM 286

Index 297

About the Author 304

acknowledgments

No doubt you have heard the cliché "There is no *I* in the word *Team.*" In a more positive sense, I would like to acknowledge the book team by saying there is definitely an *A* in this book's Team—the *A* as in *appreciate*.

I use the word appreciate in two ways. First of all, I sincerely appreciate all the hard work and dedication by the members of this book project. In another and more important sense, *appreciate* means to increase in value. By the efforts of this book team, my own knowledge of sports medicine and that of our readers has appreciated.

Special Acknowledgment: This book was inspired by my chance meeting with John Loliet, coordinator of Pinnacle Peak Park and Trail in Scottsdale, Arizona. John had spotted my Green Bay Packer shirt as I was hiking there. As an avid Packer fan, he approached me. When he heard that I was involved in sports medicine, he invited me to give a lecture at the park titled "Healthy Hiking." That seed developed and grew to become this book.

This book is about understanding, preventing, and treating outdoor recreational activities. We will focus on the following activities:

- Hiking
- Backpacking
- Road biking (paved bicycling)
- Mountain biking (dirt roads and singletrack)
- Trail running
- Rock climbing
- Mountaineering (alpine)
- Paddling (canoeing, kayaking, sea kayaking, etc.)
- Surfing
- Skiing and snowboarding (includes cross-country, backcountry, telemark, and downhill)

These outdoor recreational activities can cause "overuse" injuries. This is in contrast to ball sports (football, basketball, tennis, soccer, etc.), which cause impact and twisting injuries. This book will focus on overuse injuries. However, twisting injuries will also be presented, because they can also occur in slips and falls in running, biking, skiing, and climbing.

In 1991, I published a sports medicine book titled *Play Healthy, Stay Healthy*. Many of the thoughts and diagrams from that book will be used in this book, along with updated medical information for the fitness enthusiast. Additional chapters will be presented by medical and fitness experts.

10-Point Treatment Plan

The 10-Point Treatment Plan explained in this book evolved in response to such questions as these:

- How much activity can I have?
- What else can I do?
- Should I apply heat or cold?
- What are the appropriate exercises for injury rehabilitation?
- What medications should I use?
- What kind of diet should I be on, and what should I drink?

- What is the best outdoor shoe (and other apparel)?
- Should I use a brace?
- Should I use a walking pole?

Icons are used to illustrate three activity levels that can be applied to recreational injuries.

STOP means avoid hard use. Reduce activity.	**YIELD** means be cautious. Let pain be your guide.	**GO** means full use is fine. Listen to your body.

This icon key is applied to specific fitness injuries. The 10-Point Treatment Plan, based on commonly accepted sports medicine practice, is presented in a unique format that is easy to follow and remember. The plan explains a theory of managing injuries that includes the appropriate activity level for different kinds of outdoor recreational injuries.

With this plan, you can learn to listen to your body and establish the best activity level for your injury. Advice is based on the assumption that the most important first step for an injury is to get a correct diagnosis from a health professional. Once you have a correct diagnosis of your problem and a treatment plan, the 10-Point Treatment Plan presented here will put you back on your fitness program.

History

In the 1950s and '60s, with the growth of television coverage, recreational and competitive sports activities became extremely popular. Spurred by Dr. Ken Cooper's book *Aerobics* (1968), aerobic sports—hiking, running, swimming, and biking—became favorite worldwide activities, and not just for experienced athletes.

In 1972, Americans were inspired by the victory of marathon runner Frank Shorter in the Munich Olympics. The interest in fitness exploded. By the late '70s, the number of runners in the United States alone reached twenty million, with many thousands running marathons. Along with this activity, though, came an inevitable increase in injuries and the subsequent development of the specialty sports medicine.

Beginning in the 1980s, athletes embraced the credos "No pain, no gain" and "Winning is everything." As the intensity of workouts and competition increased, significant injury patterns emerged among fitness enthusiasts. In casual conversation and in the media, we started to hear about "tennis elbow" and "runner's knee." "Athletic highs" were sometimes replaced by "runner's depression."

Today athletes, fitness enthusiasts, and coaches are embracing the credos "Listen to your body" and "Let pain be your guide." In this book, a key aspect of the newest training and rehabilitation techniques is moderation. Derived from the Latin word *moderatus*, *moderation* means to limit extremes; think of the moderator who brings together divergent sides in a conversation. Too much of anything is not good—too much activity is just as bad as too much rest.

Organization

This book is organized in a straightforward, easy-to-use format. A standard table of contents outlines the book's topics as well as conditions may affect various body parts and where in the book to turn for advice.

Part I discusses how to respond to your body's signals and answers basic questions: Why should I listen to my body? How should I listen? To whom should I listen?

Part II introduces the treatment concepts of this book. After briefly discussing causes and types of outdoor recreational injuries, this section describes the STOP, YIELD, GO approach to activity levels for different injuries. In general, it explains the 6-Point Condition Summary and describes the 10-Point Treatment Plan that is applied in Part III.

Part III presents 40 Specific Outdoor Recreational Injury Treatments for conditions experienced frequently. These conditions are organized by body part in roughly a head-to-toe manner. Each condition illustrates the injured body part, lists the specific 6-Point Condition Summary, lists the specific 10-Point Treatment Plan, and indicates the recommended activity level.

Part IV, written by Erin Doxtator, MPT, LAT, presents thirteen specific rehabilitation exercise programs that are cross-referenced in Part III.

Part V is an important section, covering the prevention of injuries. Written by experts on nutrition, walking poles, and trail hazards, the articles here will help readers rebound from an injury and continue some level of activity.

Part VI includes a series of chapters on specific surgical procedures for those few who fail to respond to conservative treatment and want to return to hiking, running, swimming, climbing, or other outdoor recreational activities. These are written by my associates at the Sports Medicine and Orthopedic Surgery Center in Milwaukee.

Disclaimer: You should note that the medical information and advice in this book is presented only as a guide—it should be used only in conjunction with the advice of your physician or health care provider.

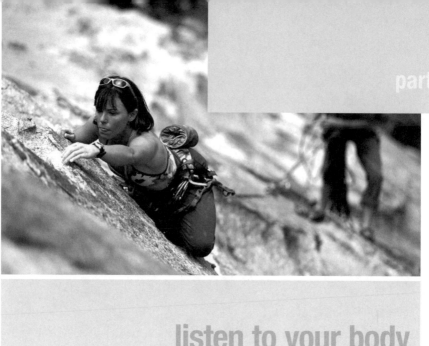

listen to your body

In outdoor recreation, too much activity can be as detrimental as too little. Part I explores not only the rewards of regular exercise but also the potential risks associated with certain outdoor activities. You can learn to balance and moderate your exercise needs. The answer is simple—listen to your body. Whenever joint and muscle problems develop, your body communicates with you through such symptoms as pain, swelling, stiffness, noise, and instability. These symptoms can come from many sources and should signal you that irritation and injury are occurring.

The following questions are answered in Part I:

- Why is it important to listen to your body?
- How does your body communicate with you?
- Who can you turn to for professional help?
- What can you expect to receive from your physician or health care provider?
- What information can you bring to your health care provider?

Why Listen to Your Body?

Athletes around the world who have experienced a sports injury immediately look outside themselves for a solution to their concerns, but their first step should really be looking and listening to their own bodies. Your body is talking to you—are you listening? Your body is telling you that there are wonderful rewards and some risks when you exercise regularly. By learning how to interpret your body's signals, you can work with your health care provider to design a treatment program that will respond precisely to your body's needs.

Participating in outdoor recreational activities is similar to investing money. You can put your money in a savings account that pays 1 percent, receive little reward, and have a low risk. Or you can purchase volatile options in the futures market, which can pay tremendous sums, but you risk losing all your money. Somewhere in between, the cautious investor buys stocks and bonds for long-term growth and stability.

Most of us seem to understand the concept of money management but have trouble understanding "body management" when it comes to choosing activities. The risks of poor money management are sometimes very clear—bankruptcy, poverty, extreme loss. We sometimes forget the risks of poor body management. We rarely think about the possibility of pain and disability that may accompany sports injuries unless an injury occurs.

Reward/Risk Ratio

Although you are involved in outdoor recreational activities because you know some of the potential rewards, occasionally reminding yourself of these rewards may keep you motivated. The rewards of outdoor recreational activities are many:

- Prevention of musculoskeletal injuries by maintaining muscle tone
- Improved flexibility and range of motion
- Prolonged physical and mental health
- Improved cardiovascular endurance
- Improved positive feeling of "good health"
- Opportunity to learn new skills
- Opportunities for friendship and socialization
- The fun of games
- Team membership
- For a few, a professional career

This list can go on, but it helps explain why sports are such an important part of our culture. Yet we sometimes lose sight of the fact that millions of people become injured and that some injuries lead to complications, even though most injuries are minor. Some of the specific complications that may result are minor musculoskeletal injury followed by a brief period of disability; major bone and joint injury, which may lead to chronic pain or arthritis; financial losses because of time spent recuperating and because of medical expenses; and mental depression, which occasionally may become severe.

You, the athlete, must decide whether the rewards of your particular outdoor recreational activity outweigh the potential risks. The younger athletes sometimes have a hard time with balancing rewards and risks because they tend to focus on the rewards and deny the risks. Because of their experience, older

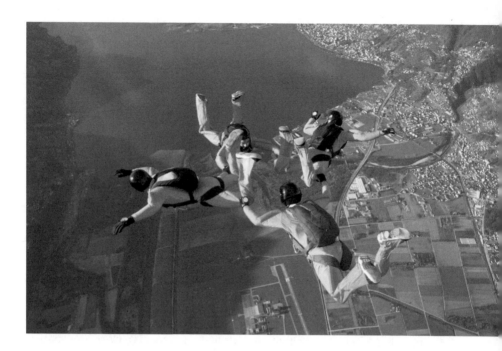

athletes are more aware of risks and approach the rewards more realistically.

Complications develop with the extremes. Too much running, biking, hiking, and climbing activities may result in injuries leading to some of the problems mentioned earlier, while inactivity can lead to:

- Weight gain
- Loss of muscle mass
- Loss of bone strength (particularly in women, who are prone to developing osteoporosis)
- Mental inactivity leading to depression
- Loss of cardiovascular conditioning

Mature judgment can lead to the appropriate level of outdoor recreational activity.

It is no surprise that young athletes in particular are confused by these potential risks and rewards associated with too much or too little activity. Achieving balance is the goal, but how? The answer is simple—just listen to your body.

Our bodies have evolved with a wonderful mechanism for letting us know when we are experiencing too much activity—in a word, pain. If you are experiencing increasing aches and discomfort in a muscle or joint, your body is telling you to moderate, reduce activities, rest a while, and change your activity.

The worst thing you can do is ignore the pain. This will only aggravate the problem and cause increasing difficulty with healing. How to deal with this pain will be explained more in Part II.

Why Exercise?

Athletes should realize that every activity has a reward/risk ratio. Generally in life, the greater the reward, the greater the risk. The faster you run or bike, the more likely you will be injured. A key lesson is understanding why you exercise. Younger athletes generally focus on the competitive aspects of sports activity, specifically on winning. Winning is part of competition. Football legend Vince Lombardi said, "Winning isn't everything—it's the only thing!" This generally reflects the viewpoint of highly competitive professional athletes. At the professional sports level, with billions of dollars at risk, winning is certainly everything. This emphasis on winning is transmitted to most athletes, even those not involved in professional competition, and can eventually lead to musculoskeletal injuries.

Unless you are a professional athlete, though, you may discover more benefits in exercising if you focus on factors other than winning, factors such as having fun and becoming physically fit. It is amazing how cautious you will become after you have experienced your first sports injury. Once you learn to listen to your body and become aware of the signals your body gives, you will be able to avoid many potentially serious injuries and successfully manage injuries once they occur.

How to Listen to Your Body

Just as with most new activities, learning how to listen to your body takes experience and practice; however, once you learn how to understand what your body is telling you, it becomes easier all the time. After all, no one knows your body better than you do.

Your body communicates with you in various ways when joint and muscle problems develop. Pain, swelling, stiffness, noise, and instability are the most common ways your body tells you that something is wrong. Let's look at these symptoms in more detail so you will be aware of them when they occur.

Pain

Think of pain as simply your body's way of telling you that injury and irritation are occurring. Pain can come from many sources. It may be due to a buildup of chemicals (such as lactic acid) to stimulate certain nerve fibers in the muscles. Pain may be due to a mechanical cause, such as general wear and tear on the body, or it can be caused by inflammation or irritation of the lining of a joint. Whatever the cause, there are basically three types of pain: vague, localized, and delayed. These types are explained more fully in Part II under "Activity Levels" (point 1 of the 10-Point Treatment Plan).

Swelling

Swelling is the accumulation of fluid around or inside a joint or muscle. That is the body's initial way of healing and is also known as the inflammatory process. The body is trying to bring blood products and fluid to fight the injury and cleanse the injured area. Sometimes the swelling and the inflammation process cause more problems than the initial injury; however, keep in mind that some swelling is necessary for healing to take place. For practical purposes, consider that a little swelling might be fine, while too much is not good and should be suppressed with anti-inflammatory treatment. Ways to treat swelling will be discussed in the 10-Point Treatment Plan section.

Stiffness

Stiffness can come from inside a joint and can be due to swelling, a torn cartilage, or arthritic spurs in a joint. Stiffness can also be caused by factors outside the joint; inflamed or tight muscles or tendons are frequent sources of such stiffness. Generally, stiffness without local pain in the joint is probably a result of muscle injury or muscle inflammation and does not imply a serious problem. Stiffness associated with local pain, though, implies a more serious condition.

Noise

Noise or snaps in the joint can be very confusing in running, biking, hiking, and climbing. Listening to noises and interpreting them correctly is very important. If the noise or snap is associated with local pain, this generally indicates a potential problem. Noise can be caused by a roughness of the joint surfaces known as chondromalacia or by an irritation of the joint associated with osteoarthritis or torn meniscus; however, in the hip or ankle, the noise can be produced by simple movement of a normal tendon gliding over a normal bony protrusion and causing a snap.

As a rule of thumb, you should moderate those activities that cause a joint to snap. Even if there is no initial pain, persistent snapping and irritation can lead to roughness and eventually tendinitis. If the joint produces a noise but no pain, stiffness, or swelling, then the noise generally can be monitored without any major change in activity; moderation is the key.

Instability

Joints are held together with muscles and ligaments. Some joints, such as the shoulders and the knees, are inherently unstable. Other joints, such as the hips, are much more stable. Joint instability or "giving way" can be the result of two different problems. One involves the internal knee joint or ligaments inside or

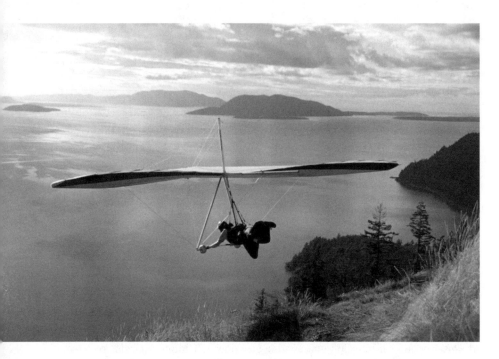

around the knee, for example, the anterior cruciate ligament. The other problem may involve factors in the muscles around the joint, for example, a weak thigh, which causes the knee to give way.

Giving way and instability can be serious problems and should not be ignored, especially by mountain climbers. Giving way, even without pain, should be carefully assessed by a health care provider. At first, instability should be treated by simply restricting those activities that cause it, working on building muscles around the joint, and carefully evaluating and treating the joint factors, such as a torn ligament or a loose fragment in the joint.

Whom to Listen To

As much as you need to be responsible for your own well-being, you also need to be able to work with health care professionals who have the experience and knowledge to guide you in the right direction. There are many health care providers who can help you, including physicians and other professionals who practice the specialty of sports medicine. With so many specialists and so much help available, the injured athlete and consumer can be very confused. When you are injured, whom should you contact for help?

Sources of Help

The chart below lists various health care professionals and other providers of help and their special expertise and skills.

Health Care Provider	Definition
Medical doctors	MDs, physicians who practice family medicine, internal medicine, general surgery, and orthopedic surgery. They are trained in medical diagnosis and treatment.
Orthopedic surgeons	MDs who are trained specifically in injuries of the musculoskeletal system; team physicians of most major sports are orthopedic surgeons. Orthopedic surgeons in the past treated the musculoskeletal deformities specifically of children. Now they treat injuries in athletes.
Osteopaths	DOs, doctors of osteopathy. Osteopaths' philosophy of medicine is based on the theory that the body is capable of making its own remedies against disease when it is in a normal structural relationship. Chief emphasis is on the importance of normal body mechanics and manipulative methods.
Podiatrists	DPMs, doctors of podiatric medicine, who specialize in care of the foot and associated injuries. Highly specialized surgical procedures are done in conjunction with orthopedic surgeons.
Chiropractors	DCs, doctors of chiropractic medicine, which is based on the theory that health and disease are related to the function of the nervous system. Diagnosis is done by identifying the irritants, and treatment is done by conservative manipulative and massage techniques. Some athletes find chiropractors very helpful in treating muscular injuries, though it is very unusual for a chiropractor to be the primary team physician for a high school, college, or professional team.
Nurses	RNs, registered nurses, health care providers who work in close conjunction with physicians and hospitals to rehabilitate and treat injured athletes.
Physical therapists	PTs, allied health professionals who deal with the diagnosis, treatment, and prevention of disease with the aid of physical agents such as light, heat, cold, water, and mechanical apparatus for musculoskeletal rehabilitation. Physical therapists work in close conjunction with physicians and orthopedic surgeons for treatment and rehabilitation. In a few select states, physical therapists are allowed to make a diagnosis and render treatment without a physician's prescription.
Trainers	ATCs, or certified athletic trainers, health professionals trained to diagnose and provide first aid on the practice

	field. They provide specialized instruction, training techniques, instruction in prevention of injuries, and immediate first aid. They work in close conjunction with physical therapists and physicians.
Coaches	The "health educators" most involved in training and rehabilitation of the athlete. At times, the coach is the first person to see the injured athlete, and coaches sometimes give advice on the management of pain.
Teachers	Frequent advisers on exercise physiology, nutrition, biology, and sports. Like coaches, teachers may walk a fine line between teaching and managing minor injuries.
Parents	Potential caretakers in educating and rendering first aid to an injured child. They can have a tremendous positive effect on guiding young athletes.
Friends	Persons often turned to for advice. Friends can be helpful in providing encouragement and in guiding you to a reliable health care provider; however, they can be the least reliable source of medical information.
You	At times the best "health care provider"—especially if you have learned the principles of this book and are able to listen to your body. Only you can fully understand your own pain level. If you learn to modify activities according to pain levels, you can be of great help to yourself in managing an injury. The 10-Point Treatment Plan outlined in this book can help you in conjunction with your doctor's diagnosis and treatment recommendations.

Obviously, there are so many possible sources of information that it can be very confusing to know where to turn for help. Who do you turn to for advice?

There are many key considerations—cost, time, and the effect on your social life and activity level. You may use this list as a guideline in sorting out alternatives for help; however, one of the best approaches is choosing a health care provider based on a reference from a friend who has had a similar problem and has been treated successfully.

The Internet has been an excellent source for athletes to find good health information about health care providers. However, the Internet can lead you through a maze of long, confusing searches. For example, a search on Google using the words *sports medicine* will produce over two million Web sites. The following Web sites are some that I recommend for patients. Their exact addresses can be found on a typical search engine such as Google or Yahoo. Here are some Internet resources for finding good health care information:

- WebMD—www.webmd.com, an excellent source of general sports medicine information.
- NOAH—www.noah-health.org, New York Online Access to Health. (This Web site is in both English and Spanish.)
- Pub Med—www.ncbi.nlm.nih.gov, National Library of Medicine.
- American Academy of Orthopaedic Surgeons—www.aaos.org.

A sports injury can be a prolonged, frustrating problem. Your first step is to listen to your body and then seek help. If your health care provider simply says, "Stop all activity, go home, and do nothing," then you may want to seek a second opinion. Keep in mind that the 10-Point Treatment Plan explained later in this book is designed to help you in conjunction with your physician's advice.

Working with Your Physician

Finding the right physician or health care provider to help you handle your injury is the first step. The next step is working well with that person so that the best results can be achieved. It is important to know how your physician organizes information and what kinds of help to expect.

If you understand how your physician organizes records, you can help organize your thoughts, and your injury management will be much more effective. You will find that most physicians use a chart to organize your medical problems into four components: subjective, objective, assessment, and plan. These important components are described here.

SUBJECTIVE

This is the history that you give the physician and includes the symptoms you perceive, for example, pain, stiffness, swelling, throbbing, or numbness. In medical school, students are taught that the history forms 85 percent of the diagnosis and is the most important aspect of the diagnosis. If you write down and organize these concerns before you see the physician, you will save time and help your physician (see Figure 1).

Injury Form

Where does your pain seem to be located?

What are the symptoms?

• Pain?
• Swelling?
• Stiffness?
• Instability?

When did these symptoms begin?

What (do you believe) caused this injury?

What activity or movement increases your pain or other symptoms?

What, if anything, have you been doing to treat this injury?

Past medical history, including dates, injuries, and previous treatments

Medication now being taken?

Any allergy to medication?

Who referred you to the physician (so a report can be sent)?

Figure 1. Form for patient to fill out before seeing a physician.

OBJECTIVE

This is what physicians perceive with their senses of sight, hearing, and touch. The physician may detect a lump, muscle atrophy, soft tissue swelling, local tenderness, or joint instability. These are all objective findings that aid in the diagnosis. Other possible objective findings come from x-rays, magnetic resonance imaging (MRI) tests, and arthrograms.

ASSESSMENT

This is the diagnosis—the physician's conclusion of what is wrong with you. An accurate assessment is derived when the physician puts together your subjective and objective findings. This is the most important reason you seek medical care: to obtain a proper diagnosis. The physician will explain to you how this conclusion is reached.

PLAN

This is the treatment program for your specific diagnosis. Part II of this book explains how an effective 10-Point Treatment Plan is organized, and Part III looks at specific treatment plans for forty common injuries.

When you consult a health care provider, you should seek an understanding of three key components: a *d*iagnosis, *o*ptions, and *c*omplications. You can remember these three words with the acronym DOC. You are probably most interested in a proper diagnosis, but you should make sure you understand your options and the possible complications of each treatment plan. If you were a patient in our office, we would advise you that ultimately you make the final decision about treatment, based on your understanding of the three key components. In bioethics, this concept is called autonomy—the right of an individual to make decisions about his or her body.

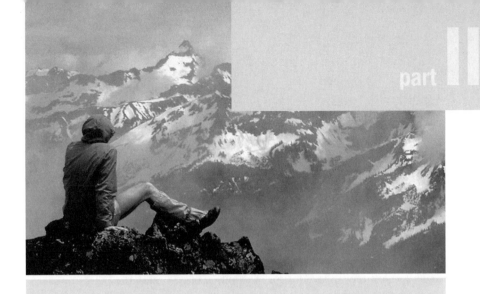

how to treat an injury

Now that you have learned to listen to your body, we will discuss the ways to treat an injury with the following:

- Identify the causes of injury
- Explain the types of injury
- Explain the STOP, YIELD, GO approach to treating injuries
- Explain the 6-Point Condition Summary for proper diagnosis
- Present the 10-Point Treatment Plan, which represents the 10 most frequent physician recommendations

The condition summary includes these six points:

1. Definition
2. Cause
3. Subjective symptoms
4. Objective findings
5. Testing procedures
6. Prognosis

The treatment plan looks at ten key aspects of treating an injury:

1. Activity levels
2. Alternative activities
3. Rehab exercises

4. Support

5. Thermal treatment

6. Medication

7. Equipment

8. Nutrition

9. Fluids

10. Surfaces

In particular, the activity level category will guide you toward the right amount of activity based on which one of three types of pain you might have: vague, localized, or delayed. Your recognition of pain underlies the STOP, YIELD, GO system to treating injuries.

What Causes Injuries?

The first step in managing injuries in outdoor recreation is preventing them in the first place, or at least lessening their severity. Knowing how to reduce your chances of suffering an injury is key to maintaining good health and to understanding sports medicine. Understanding and remembering these four factors that contribute to sports injuries can be very helpful:

- Change
- Alignment
- Twisting
- Speed

The more factors that are combined, the higher the risk for injury.

Change

The human body does not like sudden change. Overuse injuries occur when there is a sudden increase or change in training technique. Most injuries occur in spring, when there is a dramatic increase in the amount or frequency of outdoor recreation participation. Here is a good rule of thumb: Do not increase the distance, frequency, or duration of your training program by more than 10 percent a week. The human body has a wonderful adaptive power and potential—if given enough time to adapt.

Alignment

Alignment means "arrangement in a straight line." Well-aligned athletes—those born with straight legs, straight spines, and straight arms—have fewer injuries. People who have slight spine curvatures, bowed legs, or knock knees are more susceptible to injury. Young women who have wide hips and knock knees injure their kneecaps more frequently than others. Middle-aged men who become more bowlegged commonly develop knee problems. Throwing athletes, who produce more outward angulation of the arm at the elbow, are prone to elbow and shoulder injuries.

Sometimes there is little you can do if you are not born with straight alignment. In some cases, surgery can be performed to correct spinal problems, such as scoliosis, or curvature of the spine. Orthotics (arch supports) or other devices are another possibility. A podiatrist, for example, can put inserts in your shoes, which may help manage the alignment problem. The important thing to remember, if you know you have poor alignment, is to be very careful with the intensity of your approach to outdoor recreational activities. You should consult a physician about your specific concerns.

Twisting

The human body evolved primarily as a straight locomotion system for running, not for high-intensity twisting maneuvers like those performed in mountain climbing, water sports, or downhill skiing. Though twisting may help you reach your athletic goal, it also increases the likelihood that you will be injured.

Speed

When it comes to speed, the human body can be compared to a car. The more often you drive your car and the faster you drive it, the more likely it is that you will have an accident and that the accident will be serious. The faster you run, bicycle, or swim, and the more you do these activities, the more you will stress the musculoskeletal system and the more opportunity you have for injury.

The worst is a springtime athlete who, after being inactive all winter, suddenly starts exercising and has three or four factors combining to create problems. The athlete may suddenly increase the amount of exercise (change), have bowed legs (alignment), twist suddenly, and then increase speed. This athlete is very susceptible to injuries. If you are aware of these four factors, you will undoubtedly prevent most injuries from happening.

Types of Injuries

There are basically two types of injuries: acute and chronic. Using a burn as an example, you can injure yourself very badly either by putting your hand directly into a fire (resulting in an acute injury) or by overexposing yourself to the sun and burning (a chronic overuse injury). Both types of injuries can be severe and can be classified as: first, second, or third degree—third being the worst type of injury. These kinds of injuries are explained in more detail in the following sections.

Acute Traumatic Injuries

When you see a professional football player's knee being severely twisted and dislocated during a game, that is an example of an acute injury. In an acute injury, a muscle or ligament is severely torn, and a bone may be fractured. Such injuries produce a great deal of pain and swelling and require immediate first aid and referral to an emergency room.

Chronic Overuse Injuries

Most people understand the treatment procedure for an acute injury: See a doctor, rest, and avoid exercising the injured part or area. However, chronic overuse injuries in outdoor recreational activities can be just as severe but are often ignored. Stress fractures are examples of chronic overuse injuries. Fitness enthusiasts sometimes try to "run out the pain," and the result is more injury. The principle of listening to your body is very important with overuse injuries. Chronic overuse injuries are best treated by reducing activity, choosing alternative activities, treating the inflammation, if appropriate, exercising properly, and using common sense.

Reducing activities is important because the main cause of an overuse injury is usually a sudden change and then a sudden acceleration. As with a burn, reducing inflammation is one of the key treatments. You should consider applying ice, immobilizing the injured part or area, and using an anti-inflammatory medication, such as aspirin or ibuprofen. Just as we may sit in the sun and ignore the sunburn that is developing, we sometimes don't realize the extent of an injury and continue to aggravate it. When a biker or runner with a sore knee keeps pushing because the pain is minimal, problems can develop. Again, the most important principle here is to listen to your body and go with caution. There is no need to stop activity completely. Choosing alternative activities and reducing activity are just common sense.

Most outdoor recreational overuse injuries occur with twisting activities. During periods of pain, apply the STOP, YIELD, GO concept (explained in more detail in the next section) by reducing the twisting activities and progressively increasing activities that keep you moving forward, activities such as biking, running, and swimming. As pain subsides, you can gradually return to twisting endurance, strength, and speed. These factors will be explained further in Part IV.

This has been a brief summary of the types of injuries and general approaches in treating them. The 40 Specific Injury Treatments in Part III of this book will help you establish, for specific injuries, a plan using these overall concepts. The next section explains the STOP, YIELD, GO concept on which this book is based.

Stop, Yield, Go:
Learning to Listen to Your Body

In our clinic, exercise is assigned one of three activity levels and other approaches to treatment. Each of the 40 Specific Injury Treatments in Part III has a STOP, YIELD, or GO icon, which indicates the appropriate activity level. When considering activity levels, these icons are guidelines.

STOP means avoid hard use. Reduce activity.

YIELD means be cautious. Let pain be your guide.

GO means full use is fine. Listen to your body.

For instance, if your particular injury is labeled STOP, you should slow down from your normal activity level, either stopping or reducing activity almost completely. If your injury is labeled YIELD, you should be cautious about approaching outdoor recreational activities and let pain guide your level of activity. When it hurts, slow down to stop. If your activity is labeled GO, then you can pursue activity at your normal pace though you should always listen to your body for any signs of problems.

The key concept is that you should go with caution and moderation and avoid excessive pain while exercising. Identify your own strengths and weaknesses as they apply to your particular sport. For instance, if you are a mountain climber, you are probably already sufficiently flexible, but you may need work on strength. If you are a runner, you probably already have great endurance, but your performance may be enhanced by work on speed, flexibility, and strength. If you are a biker, you are already strong but may need to spend more time on endurance and flexibility. With commitment and a plan, you can balance these factors in yourself and find your activities more successful and less likely to result in injuries. Part III looks at exercise alternatives for specific injuries or conditions.

The 6-Point Condition Summary

Before considering a treatment plan, it is essential that you have a proper diagnosis from a health care professional. You should have enough information so that you can work with the professional to establish a specific treatment plan. The 40 Specific Injury Treatments in Part III of this book include a 6-Point Condition Summary. The following six points are covered for each condition:

1. Definition
2. Cause
3. Subjective symptoms
4. Objective findings
5. Testing procedures
6. Prognosis

These six points combine to give you a description of the condition, and this description is complete enough to develop a specific treatment plan.

Definition

A brief description of the key characteristics of the injury is given, including its location, anatomy, symptoms, and cause.

Cause

Medical conditions are classified by various types of causes. The first three listed here are the most common causes of outdoor recreational injuries:

Traumatic—the most frequent cause of sports injuries.

Degenerative—the middle-aged athlete is susceptible to wear and tear as the cause of pain.

Mechanical—a loose fragment in a joint could be causing pain. A pinched nerve can be from a mechanical cause.

Vascular—blood vessel block or obstruction should always be ruled out as a cause of pain in an extremity.

Tumor—a rare cause of pain in an athlete, but a tumor is one reason why an x-ray should be taken in all painful conditions.

Infection—the pain and swelling of a joint could be from infection rather than inflammation.

Psychogenic—sometimes the stress and frustration of sports cause mental discomfort.

Congenital—this is a rare but possible cause of pain in an extremity and comes from a birth defect of a bone or joint.

Metabolic—poor performance in an athlete could be from an endocrine or fluid imbalance rather than an injury.

Allergic—poor performance in sports could be from an allergy or asthma.

Subjective Symptoms

Subjective symptoms are what you as a patient perceive and should describe to your health care provider. See "Working with Your Physician" in Part I for a further description.

Objective Findings

Objective findings are what the physician perceives and detects through examination. See "Working with Your Physician" in Part I for a further description.

Testing Procedures

Testing procedures are the specialized tests that can range from simple x-rays to sophisticated surgical procedures such as arthroscopy. A list and explanations of possible tests follow.

X-rays (roentgenograms)—These "photos" are produced by an x-ray machine that takes a picture generally of a bony structure of the body. X-rays are extremely helpful in diagnosing bone injuries and fractures. They have limited value in showing soft tissue injuries in muscle, ligament, or cartilage. X-rays should be taken for almost all sports injuries to rule out congenital conditions or tumors that sometimes are masked by the sports injury.

Bone scan (radionuclide)—This test is used for the detection and localization of bone lesions and inflammation around a joint, such as arthritis. A radioactive material is injected into the bloodstream. Two or three hours later, the patient is "scanned" using a computerized sensor to measure the uptake of the material at the bone and joint level. A bone scan is a very sensitive test and is used to indicate bone turnover and reaction. A patient with a possible fracture may have a completely normal x-ray but a very "hot" bone scan.

Thermogram—This is a heat photograph using special crystal and infrared scanning equipment to measure human body surface temperature. It creates a color picture in an attempt to provide objective evidence of the pain. In our practice, we do not use therograms; however, they are available at some facilities using high-intensity computer equipment. We find thermograms of limited value.

Arthrogram—This is an x-ray study in which a radiopaque dye (which appears dense on an x-ray) is injected into the joint, generally a knee or shoulder. If there is a tear in the tendon (shoulder) or the meniscus (knee), the arthrogram can be very helpful in detecting it. The technique is technically demanding, and the results may vary with the experience of the radiologist. The MRI (see below) has essentially replaced the need for an arthrogram, except in specialized cases.

Myelogram—This form of the x-ray is taken after injecting a radiopaque material into the dural sac of the spine. This an excellent test for showing a herniated lumbar disk, but generally it is not performed unless the pain is severe and surgery is being contemplated.

MRI (magnetic resonance imaging)—This test, developed in the 1980s, produces a "photo" in response to protons and their electromagnetic force in each tissue. The result produces a significant contrast between abnormal tissue and healthy tissue. In sports injuries, an MRI is helpful in finding tears, such as of the anterior cruciate ligament, rotator cuff, or meniscus.

A retrospective literature review study was performed by our group because we have seen an increasing number of patients with a positive MRI for torn meniscus being referred for arthroscopic surgery, yet their clinical signs and symptoms do not fit that diagnosis. Fifteen orthopedic and radiology articles were found that evaluated an MRI of the knee performed on asymptomatic volunteers (people who had no knee complaints). Studies showed that patients who were older than 50 years old had as high as 40% false-positive MRIs showing a tear, yet they had no signs or symptoms of a tear. Our group shares the opinion of Drs. Bonamo and Saperstein of New York University Medical Center, who stated, "The public's growing perception of MR imaging as a near invaluable diagnostic tool and a sine qua non of surgical treatment is unfortunately often shared by the physician. As a result, MR imaging is often automatically included in every diagnostic protocol with the implicit danger that treatment will be determined primarily by the findings on the MR imaging while the patient's history, localization of symptoms and findings on physical exam are overlooked." Our orthopedic group published the study "False Positive MRI of the Knee" in the *Wisconsin Medical Journal* (2002).

CAT scan (computerized axial tomography)—Using computer-generated images, various nonsurgical "cuts"(*tomography* comes from the Greek *tomos,* meaning "section") are taken with the x-ray and integrated to produce a picture that is extremely accurate for identifying spine lesions and various bone and joint problems.

EMG (electromyogram)—This is a study of muscles used to determine various diseases or nerve and spinal injuries. Using electrical impulses, muscles are tested at rest, during voluntary contractions, and during electrical stimulation. The results help in making the proper diagnosis of a muscle or nerve injury.

EKG (electrocardiogram)—Though not specifically a test for musculoskeletal injuries, the EKG done as part of a cardiac stress test can be very helpful in an athlete's rehabilitation and for determining cardiovascular fitness.

Arthroscopy—This surgical technique, developed in the 1970s, was initially a diagnostic test to evaluate the internal structures of a joint. The procedure, now refined and performed with small scopes, can be used for the elbow and wrist. Most often this examination procedure is done under general anesthesia. Small incisions are made, and an endoscope about the diameter of a pencil, is inserted into the joint to give direct visualization of cartilage, ligaments, and meniscus lesions. This procedure is very accurate but should not be used until more traditional diagnostic techniques, such as a history and physical, routine x-rays, and perhaps an MRI, have been performed. The advantage of the arthroscopy is that after the diagnostic procedure is performed, certain surgical procedures, such as removing cartilage lesions or repairing injured ligaments, can also be performed using the arthroscope.

These tests can be expensive and confusing. However, they are helpful in integrating the history and physical examination in order to arrive at a specific diagnosis and treatment plan for an injured athlete. Your health care provider helps to correlate and integrate your history, physical condition, and diagnosis and then determines which test or tests you may need. Once these steps are completed, you are ready for a treatment plan (see the section "The 10-Point Treatment Plan").

Prognosis

Prognosis is the final step in describing a condition and providing a general guideline on what will happen as a result of a particular injury. You need to realize that medicine is not an exact science, and each case tends to act differently, though there are obvious similarities within injury categories. A health care provider does not have a crystal ball. The word *prognosis* comes from the Greek *progignōskein,* meaning "to know before." Based on the physician's experience and years of management and knowledge, the health care professional may be able to "know before" the end result actually occurs.

The 10-Point Treatment Plan

The 10-Point Treatment Plan looks at the key aspects of treating an outdoor recreational injury:

1. Activity levels
2. Alternative activities
3. Rehabilitation exercises
4. Support
5. Thermal treatment
6. Medication
7. Equipment
8. Nutrition
9. Fluids
10. Surfaces

When you are listening and then responding to your body, these items are all very important. This section will focus on each of them in detail. In Part III, specific sports injuries and conditions are explained using a 6-Point Condition Summary and then a 10-Point Treatment Plan that can be applied to each condition.

1. Activity Levels

Of the areas covered in the 10-Point Treatment Plan, activity is the most important, because it relates directly to the STOP, YIELD, GO concept. In the 40 Specific Injury Treatments, activity levels are designated by icons: STOP, YIELD and GO.

As previously discussed, you will have to learn the what, how, and who of listening for pain. There are different kinds of pain, and each warrants a different response or a different level of activity. The real dilemma in outdoor recreational injury and fitness is knowing how to differentiate among these types of pain. Activity levels in the 10-Point Treatment Plan guide you toward the right activity level based on the kind of pain you have.

STOP Avoid hard use. Reduce activity.

YIELD Let pain be your guide.

GO Listen to your body.

TYPES OF PAIN

One type of pain is vague pain, which you may experience in large muscle groups during and after exercise. This pain is probably due to a buildup of lactic acid and is a typical characteristic of a training effect. Vague pain suggests that you should reduce activities but not necessarily change your training program. In this case, YIELD, or caution, may be the most appropriate activity level. If you feel better with increasing activity, then continue with that more moderate approach.

Realize that you can be fooled and that a vague ache in your thigh may not be muscle but rather nerve pain from a herniated disk, which can be greatly aggravated by activity. If there is any question, reduce rather than increase activities. Again, here is where a diagnosis by a health care professional is very important to help you differentiate between nerve, vascular, and muscle pain. When exercising with nerve pain, it is important to concentrate on straight activities and avoid hard, sudden twisting activities.

A second type of pain is localized. It indicates a more serious problem and is located directly in the tendon, bone, joint, or ligament. You can usually put your finger right on the painful spot and say, "It hurts here." Localized pain suggests a more serious injury around the joint and probably means that your training program has gone too fast and too hard. The main treatment in this situation is a significant reduction in any outdoor recreational activities. The familiar saying "No pain, no gain" is simply *not* correct for localized pain.

One of the advantages of being an experienced athlete is that you've gone through the risks and injuries of sports and know that sometimes injuries don't completely heal, or that they take a long time to heal and lead to permanent changes in your body. The young, immature athlete doesn't have these experiences until injuries have already occurred. Some of the risks of abusing and using an inflamed, painful joint include permanent damage, such as arthritis, torn meniscus, torn tendons, and stress fractures.

The third type of pain you may encounter is delayed. When planning your activity level, you should be aware of the possibility of delayed pain such as that caused by overuse of a joint. Arthritis pain or chondromalacia of the knee doesn't give you immediate feedback. You can injure yourself but not feel it until a day or so later, and this can be frustrating. Here, careful monitoring is vital. Keep reducing activity until pain is at a minimal level. Don't exercise hard two days in a row—follow a hard day with a light day in order to give your body time to rest and recover.

2. Alternative Activities

Choosing alternative activities is an important aspect of treating most injuries. Consequently, alternative activities are an important part of any effective treatment plan. Though the best treatment for a painful joint or muscle is sometimes to stop all activities and rest completely, there are several major complications that can occur from the abrupt halt of all activities—cardiovascular deconditioning, muscle atrophy, increased body fat, mental depression, and bone loss or osteoporosis, to name a few. The secret is to treat the entire body, not just the painful area. The best treatment plan is moderation and listening to your body.

At our clinic, we classify activities as three types.

STOP Avoid hard twisting activities— basketball, volleyball, racquetball, wrestling, football, soccer

YIELD Moderate twisting activities— dancing, tennis, bowling, golf, skiing

GO Straight activities—race walking, swimming, biking, jogging, running, cross-country skiing, jumping rope

Keep in mind that another factor in these classifications is intensity. Some activities can be either high or low impact. For instance, aerobic dancing, though usually classified as a moderate, or YIELD activity, can actually be done at any of the levels, depending on the intensity of participation.

From our years of experience in treating fitness and sports injuries, we have found that competitive athletes will not accept the advice to stop all activities and rest. During the rehabilitation of any injury, a gradual, progressive increase in activity level should be permitted, starting with walking or swimming, then progressing to biking or running and eventually to the moderate twisting activities, and progressing eventually to hard twisting activities, usually ball sports or mountain climbing.

Generally, sports injuries are "sport specific"; that is, injuries occur primarily in one sport. The mountain climber tends to have a recurrence of injuries common to mountain climbing but will be able to hike or swim with minimal difficulty. Very simply, if you are having pain with one activity, switch activities. You don't necessarily have to stop all outdoor recreational activities.

There are many considerations when choosing an alternative activity. Your choice may be based in part on how competitive you are in the activity you normally pursue. Do you want to risk the deconditioning of the muscles you usually use for the sake of ongoing activity? The choice is up to you. Just be sure you consider your goals and try to stay active if that is the recommendation of your treatment plan.

3. Rehabilitation Exercises

Rehabilitation, or rehab, exercises are the specific exercises you pursue to condition your injured muscles so that you can return to your regular sport as a full participant. Rehab exercises are an integral part of a treatment plan and are in addition to any other activity or alternative activity, as explained earlier. Muscles have four important qualities (remembered as FESS), which can be enhanced with exercise:

- Flexibility

- Endurance

- Strength

- Speed

Even the best athletes who naturally have these qualities developed at a high level usually have room for improvement in one area or another.

Some athletes have great flexibility but lack endurance or strength. A marathon runner may have fantastic endurance but may lack strength and flexibility. Mountain climbers may have tremendous strength but may lack flexibility and endurance. The list of strengths and weakness can go on and on for each sport (see Table 1).

A question often arises: Which is more important, flexibility, endurance, speed, or strength? The answer is this: Only you know. Listen to your body. Ask yourself: Are you stiff? Are you weak? Are you winded? Are you slow? The goal for fitness enthusiasts and athletes is to identify their individual strengths and weaknesses, particularly as they relate to activities they would like to pursue. When areas needing improvement are identified, an exercise plan can be established. For the athlete needing work in all areas, we suggest the following order of importance: strength, endurance, flexibility, speed.

TABLE 1. QUALITIES OF MUSCLES FOR SELECTED SPORTS

Sport	Flexibility	Endurance	Strength	Speed
Cross-country skiing	+	o	o	o
Running	o	+	o	o
Swimming	o	o	+	o
Mountain climbing	+	+	+	+

+ indicates more important quality
o indicates less important quality

The guidelines for rehab exercises are as follows.

STOP Avoid a hard, bouncing stretch; avoid vigorously bent joint with weights.

YIELD Moderate stretch; moderately bent joint with weights

GO Light stretch: joint straight with weights

Flexibility training can be helpful, but it may be the area that is most often overemphasized. It is even possible to become too flexible if you go beyond the range of motion for a particular joint, opening up the possibility of more injuries. If there is any question, spend more of your time on strength than on flexibility training.

STRETCHING
An important part of any exercise or activity program is stretching. Listen to your body for indications of when to stretch. If you're feeling tight, then that is an indication that you should stretch. If you feel tight primarily before you exercise, then that is the best time to stretch. If you feel tight after you exercise, then that is the best time for you to stretch. There are specific guidelines that relate to stretching, and they are important to follow.

In our office, we more often see people who hurt themselves while stretching than while doing strengthening exercises. You should always make sure your muscles are warmed up before starting stretching exercises, but note that warming up doesn't mean stretching. It means making sure that your muscles are warm before beginning any stretching exercises. This means inducing a light sweat either by external heat (steam, hot pad, etc.) or by light activity (running, walking, etc.). Once your muscles are warm, start with static stretches, which do not go beyond the range of motion of your joints. You should hold these stretches for 6 to 8 seconds each and repeat them 3 to 10 times.

Athletes are most likely to be hurt when there is an imbalance between flexibility, endurance, strength and speed. Olympic gold medal winners, professional athletes, and world champions are blessed with high development in all these areas, but they have also learned how to balance their abilities. Your goal as a fitness enthusiast is to identify your areas of weakness and concentrate on improving those areas through proper muscle development, endurance, and aerobic training.

It takes motivation to establish a regular exercise program aimed at rehabilitating muscles and developing these four qualities. The ideal is to be self-motivated enough to train and exercise without the need of special equipment, trainers, coaches, or physical therapists. You should look for help in identifying areas for improvement and for help in providing appropriate incentives and in setting goals. Sometimes it is easier to be motivated when you are in a class or group with others who have similar goals. It is a rare person who can remain motivated all alone in a cold, damp basement while lifting weights or timing the minutes on an exercise bike. When your body tells you it needs exercise, that should be enough motivation for most committed athletes.

Controversy still exists as to whether or not stretching is effective in reducing sports injuries. A 2004 study published by Dr. Thacker and colleagues of the Centers for Disease Control and Prevention reviewed 361 scientific articles comparing stretching with other methods to prevent injury. The researchers concluded that stretching was not significantly associated with a reduction in total injuries: "There is no sufficient evidence to endorse or discontinue routine stretching before or after exercise to prevent injury among competitive or recreational athletes. . . Further research [is] recommended in well-controlled trials to determine the proper rule of stretching in sports."

EXERCISES USING EQUIPMENT

Three standard types of conditioning exercises involve equipment. Isometric refers to keeping the joint straight and adding variable resistance. An example is straight-leg-raising exercises with weights on the shin. Isometric exercises are good for situations in which full range of motion is painful.

Isotonic exercises are standard weight-lifting procedures that combine progressive resistant exercises with joint motion. Equipment includes barbells and weight machines such as the Nautilus and Universal systems. Isokinetic machines have fixed speed and a variable resistance with an accommodating resistance. An example of this type is the Cybex system typically used in a clinical setting. Isokinetic machines are excellent for rehabilitation of injured knee ligaments, such as the anterior cruciate, if no pain is produced.

The STOP, YIELD, GO concept is also applied to rehabilitation exercises. STOP means avoiding hard stretching and vigorous bent-joint activities with weights; if you are injured. YIELD means doing moderate stretching and bent-joint activities with light weights with caution after you listen to your body. GO means doing light stretching and straight-joint exercises with light weights. These should be performed early in the rehabilitation process when the joint is still sore. For example, if the ankle and knee are painful, do your exercises without moving the joint (isometric). Putting simple elastic tubing and light weights on the shin and foot will allow you to exercise joints such as the hip without experiencing pain at the ankle.

The illustrations in Part IV demonstrate how to perform many of these exercises. These exercises have been used successfully by thousands of athletes at our sports medicine clinic. In the final analysis, go with caution and moderation. Avoid exercises that cause excessive pain. Identify your own strengths and weakness as they apply to your particular sport.

4. Support

Braces, bandages, and tape around inflamed muscles and joints can be used for temporary support and stabilization. The best support, however, is your normal muscle development. If you want to build support and think you need a brace, start by developing strong muscles. Until you have proper muscle and joint stability, it is certainly advisable to wear a brace.

TYPES OF BRACES

For the knee, which is the most commonly braced joint, your choices (with approximate cost) include:

- Simple elastic bandage ($5.00)
- Elastic pull-on ($45.00)
- Neoprene elastic pull-on ($45.00)
- Knit, with metal hinges ($95.00)
- Complex patella stabilizing ($95.00)
- Semi-custom-made plastic and metal stabilizing ($500)
- Custom-made metal and plastic hinge ($850–$1,500)

The selection of a knee brace is frequently confusing for both the patent and the health care provider. Here again, listen to your body to give you guidance. If you are doing hard pivoting, twisting, and jumping activities and feel that your knee is shifting out of place, your physician may prescribe a high-tech brace for the diagnosis of a torn ligament. There is no guarantee that the brace will correct the problem, but it can be very helpful when combined with cautious exercise and adequate muscle rehabilitation. The brace may not cure you, and you may need surgery. For moderate, simple activities, a less expensive brace can certainly do the job. Many braces may be partly reimbursed by health insurance carriers if they are prescribed by a physician.

BRACES FOR EVERYONE?

As in all aspects of medicine, particular braces should be used for selected problems in certain instances. A brace should not be used as an excuse not to exercise your muscles.

One of the major advantages of a brace is that it becomes a visual symbol to others—a symbol that you have a problem. Nobody likes to admit to having a sore knee or to ask for help or less stress; however, by putting a brace on your knee or your elbow, you are saying, "Take it easy, I need help. I am listening to my body." Don't look for a "quick fix" with a brace, though. Braces are not a panacea for all joint problems. Braces, as with medications, have benefits, risks, and complications.

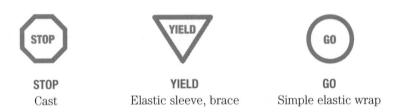

STOP	YIELD	GO
Cast	Elastic sleeve, brace	Simple elastic wrap

5. Thermal Treatment

Thermal treatment refers to the application of heat or cold to an injury. Though many first-aid manuals suggest using ice for the first 24 to 48 hours after an injury and then switching to heat, people seem to remember the word *heat* more often than *ice*. The general rule is that localized pain or any localized swelling should be treated with ice. The STOP, YIELD, and GO classifications for thermal treatment are as follows:

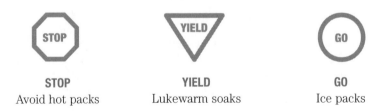

STOP	YIELD	GO
Avoid hot packs	Lukewarm soaks	Ice packs

Short of a severely dislocated joint or fractured bone, which requires emergency treatment, the initial treatment of acute traumatic injuries is reflected in the acronym RICE:

R   Rest
I   Ice
C   Compression
E   Elevation

A burn is a helpful example to illustrate the treatment of a sports injury. With an acute burn of the hand, there is an initial injury of tissue, an outpouring of fluid, and damage to the capillaries, all resulting in swelling—the inflammatory process. The initial treatment is RICE to reduce swelling and to rest tissues. Think of a sports injury as a burn. Immediately take the injured area "out of the fire," and apply ice. (More detail on ice is presented in the next section.) Rest reduces tissue damage and persistent inflammation by immobilizing the injured area. Rest can range from reduced activity to a complete immobilization of the injured part or area by, for instance, a leg cast. Compression means wrapping the injured part or area so that tissue pressure is maintained and the injured area and injured joint or muscle is immobilized. You should be careful not to apply too much compression because constriction of the blood vessels can result in vascular complications. Elevation means reducing swelling by raising the injured part or area above the heart or by simply lying down and keeping the leg or arm elevated. Elevation is appropriate during initial periods of pain and swelling.

ICE IS NICE

Ice is the key component of RICE. Ice is an extremely effective initial treatment for most outdoor recreation injuries: It acts as a local anesthetic to help relieve pain and also helps enhance the flow of blood from the skin to the deeper tissues for healing. It is a mistake, in fact, to treat an injury initially with heat because it causes more swelling and inflammation. Some trainers use the concept PIE, which stands for Pressure, Ice, and Elevation. In this approach, the previous words *rest* and *compression* are replaced with the concept of pressure. Thus, the trainer will use an iced bandage that is immediately wrapped around the injured area. The result will be a reduced outpouring of fluid—less edema.

Another effective way to use ice is in a Styrofoam cup that is filled with water, frozen, and left in a freezer. The ice in the cup (you may need to peel away some of the cup to expose the ice) can be used for a local massage for pain caused by tendinitis, tennis elbow, or ankle sprain.

Ice should be considered a medication with a prescribed dose and frequency of use. Generally, 10 or 15 minutes of an ice bath or local ice pack is all skin can tolerate. Ice can be used three or four times a day, but, as with any medication, complications may develop if it is overused.

I am reminded of the case of a basketball player who injured his ankle in a game. The coach directed him to keep his ankle in an ice bucket for 2 full days nonstop. After a while, the ice became an anesthetic, and the pain disappeared; however, the ice continued to have an effect. After 40 hours, the circulation in the player's foot stopped. Gangrene developed in the player's forefoot, and some toes had to be amputated—a tragic and definitely avoidable event. Like anything in life—and medicine—too much of a good thing can be more dangerous than the original problem.

SWITCHING FROM ICE TO HEAT

Knowing when to switch from ice to heat is based on the principle of how to listen to your body. As the local pain, tenderness, and swelling gradually subside and the symptoms change to tightness and stiffness, you can start to loosen the muscle with warm soaks and then local heat application.

Heat is good for loosening the muscles in the large muscle groups around the thigh, back, and shoulders. The general rule is to use heat before activity and ice after the activity. If you are ever in the locker room of a professional baseball team, observe the pitchers. Hot packs are applied around the shoulder and elbow for 1 to 2 hours before the game. The arm is kept warm in a thick jacket. The pitcher then performs, keeping the pitching arm warm with a jacket between innings. Immediately after the game, a trainer will put the elbow into an ice whirlpool or ice bucket to reduce pain, inflammation, and swelling.

Many people, even athletes, do not understand this principle of applying heat before and the ice or cold after the activity. For instance, at most health clubs you will see people sitting in the sauna, steam room, or hot whirlpool after a racquetball or tennis game. The process probably should be reversed. You should warm up in the sauna for about 5 minutes before an activity. Afterwards, you don't need to warm up, but that's when most people do it. Of course, you can warm up too much and find yourself exhausted before you even start to exercise. That's why 5 minutes of warm-up is usually sufficient.

For general discomfort and tightness, heat is most effective for the large muscle groups around the thigh, shoulders, back, and neck. There are no absolute rules for the application of heat, and it can be used in combination or in contrast with ice. Try 10 minutes of heat, followed by 5 minutes of ice massage, followed by another 10 minutes of heat. The contrast may alter blood flow and enhance healing.

When deciding whether to apply heat or ice, be flexible, consider various approaches, and listen to your body. If ice is not working, then switch to heat. If heat is not working, then switch to ice. Combining the two may be very effective. Always keep in mind that overdoing heat or ice may result in complications that can be worse than the original injury.

6. Medication

Medications are potentially part of most treatment plans, and they lend themselves nicely to the STOP, YIELD, and GO classifications.

STOP Avoid high doses and excessive use of medications, vitamins, or minerals.

YIELD You may take prescribed anti-inflammatory medications and possibly local steroid injections.

GO You may take over-the-counter acetaminophen (Tylenol)—two with meals.

DIFFERENT APPROACHES TO MEDICATIONS

Medications are helpful for two reasons: They relieve pain and reduce local inflammation. There are two extreme attitudes toward medications. One extreme attitude is to avoid any form of medication. The other is to look for a "quick fix" and take excessive quantities of minerals, vitamins, and anti-inflammatory medication in hopes of curing the condition. The cautious approach is one of moderation and listening to your body, which might include taking minimal doses of anti-inflammatory medication.

As with most aspects of a treatment plan, there are problems with either extreme. You may experience complications by not taking medication when it is warranted; however, you will also experience complications by taking excessive medications. Sometimes a little bit of help in the form of pain and anti-inflammatory relief is needed during the rehabilitation process, but somewhere you need to find a happy medium. This can usually be accomplished by letting your body indicate what medication produces the best results and can be tolerated. There are no fixed rules when it comes to medications.

ANTI-INFLAMMATORY AND OVER-THE-COUNTER MEDICATIONS

Nonsteroidal, anti-inflammatory drugs act by changing the local chemistry at the inflamed site through various modes of action. A full discussion of medications is beyond the scope of this book. Most of the strong anti-inflammatory medications can have major side effects: gastrointestinal upset and heart disease. We tell patients that one in one hundred patients on these medications may develop a gastric ulcer. You must balance the rewards of taking medication with the potential complications and risks. Again, the principle is to listen to your body.

In recent years a new classification of medications called COX inhibitors, or "coxibs" were introduced. These medications inhibited the synthesis of prostaglandin via the inhibition of an enzyme, cyclooxygenase-2 (COX-2). Known by the brand names Vioxx and Celebrex, they caused less stomach upset, but they were expensive and required a physician's prescription.

In 2005 the Federal Drug Administration issued prescription warnings for Celebrex, Bextra, and Vioxx because of cardiovascular complications. Thus, for my patients with injuries from recreational activities, I recommend acetaminophen (Tylenol) as the initial medication of choice because of its fine safety record.

ANTI-INFLAMMATORY INJECTION

The product we use in our office is called Kenalog. It is a crystal steroid product related to cortisone. Cortisone is a naturally occurring substance made in the body to help fight stress and inflammation and to promote healing. The medication helps to relieve local inflammation such as tendinitis, synovitis, and localized arthritis. Occasionally, the injection is used as a "test" for inflammation versus mechanical tear. If the pain rapidly subsides and is relieved, the pain was probably from an inflammation. If pain persists, the pain may be from a mechanical tear.

The mechanism of action or how the injection works is to reduce inflammation, promote healing, and decrease scar formation. A possible side effect in a dark-skinned person may be local depigmentation and whitening of the skin. There may be a temporary weakening of the injected tendon. Therefore, caution in hard jumping is recommended for about 2 to 4 weeks after the injection.

Local pain and swelling sometimes follow the injection. If there is a local flare-up, you should limit activity, and you may apply ice and take Tylenol for 1 or 2 days. Anti-inflammatory injections should not be abused and should not be a substitute for common sense and modification of activity. As with all medications, there are risks and rewards, and you should discuss them with your physician. In our practice, we have found that one local injection of steroid in and around an inflamed joint that has not responded to treatment is a safe approach compared with the potential complications of more aggressive treatment such as surgery.

7. Equipment

As part of rehabilitation or training, exercise equipment is very important for cardiovascular and musculoskeletal development. The list of possible equipment you can buy includes treadmill, cross-country ski machine, bicycle, stair-climbing apparatus, rowing machine, and weight-lifting equipment (free weights and isotonic machines). Other equipment is available for purchase; however, these are the most common and the most useful pieces of equipment available.

Patients and athletes are frequently overwhelmed by the multitude of equipment. Your decision depends on many factors—availability, cost, space, and personal objectives and motivation. Here again, the principle of listening to your body should dictate which equipment to buy; however, there are other alternatives to buying expensive equipment. One is to join a health club, where all of this equipment is there for you to use. You can also perform many effective exercises yourself with such simple materials as sandbags and rubber tubing. The treatment plan that has evolved for many patients in our clinic includes the use of free weights—sandbags of 3, 5, and 10 pounds that can be applied to the arm or leg for strength training. Rubber tubing can be used for flexibility training and strengthening.

The STOP, YIELD and GO classifications for equipment are as follows:

STOP Avoid vigorous stair climbing. Avoid strenuous weight lifting.

YIELD Rowing, moderate weight lifting

GO Treadmill, bike, cross-country skiing

EQUIPMENT CHOICES

The following explanations are based on the assumption that you are planning to buy equipment for your home and that you need to make the right choices.

Treadmills. Since the 1980s, the cost of electric treadmills has gradually come down, to between $500 and $1,000. Some very sophisticated treadmills can cost between $3,000 and $5,000, but these are generally not necessary for the average athlete. Certain considerations are weight, noise, and ability to change incline and speed. At about the $1,000 range, an electric treadmill can give you many of the features and running durability that you need.

Even though running on a treadmill seems to simulate normal running or walking, it is not the case. The tread is moving rapidly against your foot. This can sometimes aggravate minor pain around the front of the knee in the region of the patella. The aggravation is generally brief but is a reason to go slowly and moderately. During your first few days with the equipment you may tend to push yourself as hard as possible and ignore minor problems. This can lead to endless frustration from pain, and eventually you stop using your $1,000 toy.

Cross-country ski machine. An indoor cross-country ski machine has been available for many years. Several inexpensive copies of the original have become available. Just as cross-county skiing provides excellent upper- and lower-body exercise, so do cross-country machines. Sometimes the twisting of the upper body can produce low back and neck discomfort.

Bicycle. Stationary bicycles have been available for many years. One of the concerns is that they are too upright and do not have the same handlebar-to-seat alignment ratios as a regular outdoor touring bicycle. An approach to this problem is to take a mountain bike and purchase a wind trainer, which is a stand to put on the rear wheel for home use. This gives you the best of both worlds. You have a year-round bicycle for outdoor biking and indoor biking at a moderate price. This way you are assured of having an indoor bicycle that fits your body frame.

Many of the bicycles at clubs, even though they are adjustable, are rarely adjusted to your body size. This is a frequent cause of neck, back, and knee complaints in the club bicyclist. Other indoor bicycle alternatives feature a large oscillating fan on the front wheel. This large front wheel is also controlled by reciprocally moving handlebars. This gives you the ability to exercise both your arms and your legs at the same time. An advantage is that you can still exercise your upper body yet also rest and protect a painful knee and ankle if necessary.

Rowing machines. Rowing machines have been very popular for the last 20 years. One of the most popular features a large flywheel, which produces wind resistance and excellent cooling for the rower. Excessive knee bending and back flexion can occur with rowing; rowing should, therefore, be used in moderation for patients with knee and back problems.

Elliptical trainer. This hybrid machine mimics the movements of the knee, similar to a bicycle and a treadmill combined, and it operates in a vertical position. Theoretically, there is less stress on the knee; however, some patients experience increased pain about patella.

Weight-lifting equipment. The weight lifter has two choices: either free weights or isotonic weight machines. In our clinic, we start patients with simple 5- to 10-pound sandbags that can be wrapped around the calf, thigh, or arm to gradually build up flexibility, endurance, speed, and strength (see previous section, "Rehabilitation Exercises"). From free weights, you can progress to dumbbells, which may have some advantages over machines. Dumbbell weights help you learn to coordinate your muscles with added balance and resistance, while the isotonic machines (Universal, Nautilus) offer excellent resistance through the full range of motion but do not help with coordination and balance. The machine weights can especially aggravate any patellar problems because of the added resistance when the knee is flexed. The rule here is to go gradually and moderately and avoid excessive flexion. Listen to your body. If pain is developing around the joint, change the routine to other joints. "Circuit training" is an excellent aerobic exercise in which you move from station to station perhaps every 5 minutes so that you change resistance and wear on any specific joint area.

CHOOSING SHOES

Shoes are undoubtedly the most important piece of equipment an outdoor recreational enthusiast can buy; yet, for the serious runner and athlete, nothing is more confusing and frustrating than trying to find and buy shoes. Try to find a truly knowledgeable shoe salesperson who participates in your specific activity (running, biking, climbing, and so forth). Guidelines for choosing athletic shoes are actually very simple. See the chapter by Dr. Thomas A. Pietrocarlo in Part VI of this book for further discussion about shoes and foot problems.

Avoid testimonials. Most of us buy running shoes because of the hard sell from TV and magazine commercials with testimonials. The shoe industry is a multi-billion-dollar industry with high profits and high-paid testimonials, which are probably the least reliable source of information for the serious consumer. Very little scientific information is presented to help the consumer make an intelligent choice. Shoes have been promoted for their softness, air, gel, and shock absorption; shoe companies have discovered that this is the best way to sell merchandise. Avoid the trap of buying a shoe simply because a world-class athlete uses it.

Avoid "cheap skates." The term *cheap skates* means exactly that. Inexpensive skates are bad for skating, and inexpensive shoes are bad for running and walking. One of your best protections is to buy the top-of-the-line model. Some manufactures sell very expensive shoes to promote their name but also have very cheap models with a famous logo. Be careful of a cheap shoe with a fancy name.

Buy a shoe that fits. The first step in purchasing athletic shoes of any kind is deciding whether you will buy a straight or a curved last. The last is the sole of the shoe. A curved last encourages pronation, while a straight last resists it. Pronation is the lowering or rolling-in motion of the inner, long arch of the foot, forming a flat foot. European shoes tend to be very narrow and straight, while American shoes tend to be somewhat wider and curved. In the early 1980s, many shoes had a curved last. Since then, studies have shown that during running the foot straightens, so you should have more of a straight shoe. So, if your sport involves running, a straight shoe will be best.

If you are not sure what shape foot you have, try moving fast (run) while barefoot on a wet surface that will take an impression. If your footprint curves inward, then buy a curved-last shoe. If your footprint is straight, then buy a straight-last shoe. Look at your footprint while walking and running. Generally, your walking footprint curves in, while the running footprint is straighter.

Buy a shoe for comfort and protection. Many shoes now are marketed for shock absorption, but we have found that shock-absorption shoes are not stable enough and do not give you the protection and rear foot control needed for most outdoor recreational activities. You should avoid shoes that are promoted for "performance" or "speed." It is highly unlikely that you will perform and run faster because of your shoe. You need a shoe for protection.

Choose a shoe for the right features. The right features are these:

- Forefoot flexibility—The normal foot flexes easily at the metatarsal region. Look at your foot and flex your toes, and you will see the forefoot creases. A good shoe will move like the normal foot. Inexpensive children's shoes are built on a board with very poor flexibility. Adults don't tolerate that rigid shoe and develop foot, ankle, and knee problems.

- Torsional (twisting) stability—Inexpensive shoes are either too rigid or too flexible when twisted. A good test is to take a running shoe and twist it as if you were squeezing a rag. It should resist the twisting and have a good torsional stability for good control of your foot.

- Firmer heel control—A sign of a poorly built shoe is a very flexible heel counter (the firm back area around the heel) with very poor support, such as what you would find in a bedroom slipper that has a soft heel and no counter. The more money you put into the shoe, the firmer the heel control becomes. This is a sign of a good shoe.

8. Nutrition

In December 1984, the National Institutes of Health made a strong statement recommending that Americans lower the fat and cholesterol content of their diets. It was recommended that the average athlete who is at an appropriate weight should maintain a diet that provides about 30 percent calories from fat. An excellent source of nutrition information is the National Institutes of Health Web site, www.nih.org. A more comprehensive discussion on the nutritional needs for outdoor activities is provided in Part V of this book.

STOP 45 percent of diet is fat calories— U.S. diet

YIELD 30 percent of diet is fat calories— heart disease diet

GO 15 to 20 percent of diet is fat calories— low-fat diet

SERUM CHOLESTEROL AND ACTIVITY

How activity affects cholesterol levels is of particular interest to the athlete. Our clinic conducted a study of 500 patients undergoing arthroscopic surgery. A serum blood cholesterol test was performed just prior to surgery. The results were published in the *American Medical Athletic Association Newsletter,* (April 1998).

A positive correlation was found between those patients having chondromalacia (osteoarthritis) and elevated serum cholesterol. A serum cholesterol over 200 may be one of the risk factors associated with wear and tear of the joints. These preliminary findings may suggest that an elevated serum cholesterol may be a metabolic or vascular factor associated with the development of osteoarthritis.

The serum cholesterol test helps us differentiate between "healthy" and "fit" patients. The untimely death of marathon runner and author Jim Fixx reminds us that seemingly fit runners may not be as healthy as they appear. Fixx, who died unexpectedly following a run, had a cholesterol level of 250 milligrams. An autopsy revealed that besides extensive arteriosclerotic heart disease, he had an acute myocardial infarction.

In April 2005 the U.S. Agricultural Department revised its 1992 food pyramid. It now emphasizes physical activity—30 minutes a day—with low-fat recommendations (www.mypyramid.gov).

9. Fluids

Proper hydration (drinking enough water) is one of the few areas in sports medicine where listening to your body does not work. If you wait until you are thirsty, it's probably too late. You're already dehydrated. It is extremely important to drink early and plentifully during exercise. A helpful principle is "a pint a pound, the world around," meaning that for every pound you lose, you must drink a pint of water (two 8-ounce glasses). It is beyond the scope of this book to discuss in depth the exercise physiology of dehydration and water needs. Suffice it to say that your cardiovascular system and your musculoskeletal system cannot work properly unless they have adequate fluid and electrolyte balance.

The STOP, YIELD, and GO classifications for fluid are as follows:

STOP Avoid high salt, high sugar   **YIELD** Low salt, low sugar, low caffeine   **GO** Water is best

WATER: THE BEST DRINK OF ALL

The most important beverage to drink is water. There are two considerations when taking fluids: water and salt. The more poorly conditioned you are, the more salt you will lose. Therefore, early in your training, it is certainly advisable to add some salt to your fluids. There is no need to buy commercially prepared drinks that are costly and perhaps do not have the exact formula your body needs. Certain fluid supplements have alcohol and caffeine, which certainly give you a "high" but can also cause you to urinate and become more dehydrated as you urinate more. Water is the best drink.

Science so far has not developed the perfect drink for all athletes. The more you train, the more you will learn what to drink. The best advice is to listen to your body to determine what beverage, and how much, is best. If you're interested in a drink other than water, a safe and moderate approach would be to purchase some of the commercially prepared drinks aimed at athletes and dilute them 25 to 50 percent. Don't be impressed by the commercials and endorsements, which can be misleading, exaggerated, and even untrue.

Can you drink too much water? The answer is, "Yes." A scientific study published in the *New England Journal of Medicine* in April 2005 focused on hyponatremia among runners in the Boston Marathon. Hyponatremia, a low blood sodium level, was found in 13 percent of the runners at the finish line of the 26.2-mile marathon. This accounted as an important cause of race-related death and life-threatening illness among long-distance runners. The study found that those with hyponatremia has substantial weight gain, drank more than 3 liters of fluids during the race, drank fluids every mile, and had a racing time of more than 4 hours. Weight gain was the important sign of this condition.

Thus an important message of this book is moderation. The vital message of the Boston Marathon study is that moderation also applies to your fluid intake.

10. Surfaces

Of all treatment points, this may be one of the most ignored by outdoor fitness enthusiasts. Yet the surface you hit has a major impact on your body. A surface can either discourage or encourage injuries. There is a wide range of possible surfaces for athletic competition; however, they can be divided into three basis types:

STOP Avoid concrete

YIELD Blacktop streets, indoor tracks (16 or fewer laps per mile)

GO Blacktop bicycle paths, or indoor paths (8 to 10 laps per mile)

CONCRETE AND WOOD

It is best to avoid these hard surfaces as much as possible. These surfaces don't "give" and thus can intensely jar the body on impact, resulting in serious injuries. Jokingly, a good rule of thumb is not to run on anything you wouldn't pound your head on.

Careful attention should be paid to surfaces for indoor high- and low-impact aerobics. Suspended wood surfaces such as what dancers would choose are best for these activities. You should avoid working out on carpeted surfaces with concrete underneath.

BLACKTOPS, BICYCLE PATHS, INDOOR PATHS

For running and biking, a blacktop bicycle path is one of the best surfaces. Be very careful with indoor tracks that require more than 16 laps per mile. These will cause excessive twisting, turning, and stress to the ankle, knee, hip, and back.

Summary

The STOP, YIELD, GO approach (using the STOP, YIELD, and GO icons) for each of the points within the 10-Point Treatment Plan are summarized below:

1. Activity Levels

     Avoid hard use. Reduce activity.

     Let pain be your guide.

     Full use; listen to your body.

2. Alternative Activities

     Avoid hard twisting activities—basketball, volleyball, racquetball, wrestling, football, soccer.

     Moderate twisting activities—dancing, tennis, bowling, golf, skiing.

     Straight activities—race walking, swimming, biking, jogging, running, cross-country skiing, jumping rope.

3. Rehabilitation Exercises

STOP Avoid a hard, bouncing stretch; avoid vigorously bent joint with weights.

YIELD Moderate stretch; moderately bent joint with weights.

GO Light stretch: joint straight with weights.

4. Support

STOP Cast.

YIELD Elastic sleeve, brace.

GO Simple elastic wrap.

5. Thermal Treatment

STOP Avoid hot packs.

YIELD Lukewarm soaks.

GO Ice packs.

6. Medication

STOP Avoid high doses and excessive use of medications, vitamins, or minerals.

YIELD You may take prescribed anti-inflammatory medications and possibly local steroid injections.

GO You may take over-the-counter medications such as Tylenol—two with meals.

7. Equipment

STOP Avoid vigorous stair climbing. Avoid strenuous weight lifting.

YIELD Rowing, moderate weight lifting.

GO Treadmill, bike, cross-country skiing.

8. Nutrition Recommended (percent of fat calories)

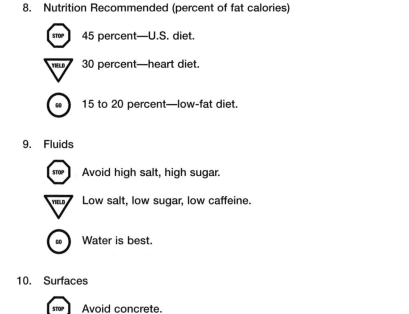

STOP   45 percent—U.S. diet.

YIELD   30 percent—heart diet.

GO   15 to 20 percent—low-fat diet.

9. Fluids

STOP   Avoid high salt, high sugar.

YIELD   Low salt, low sugar, low caffeine.

GO   Water is best.

10. Surfaces

STOP   Avoid concrete.

YIELD   Blacktop streets, indoor tracks (16 or fewer laps per mile).

GO   Blacktop bike paths, or indoor tracks (8 to 10 laps per mile).

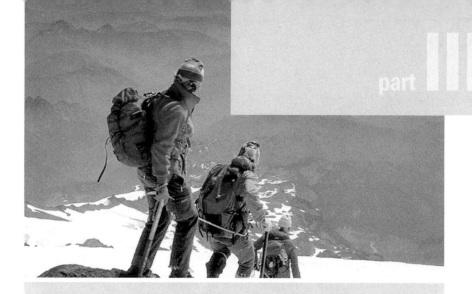

part III

40 specific outdoor recreational injuries and treatments

You can locate a specific injury in Part III in four ways: (1) See the general head-to-toe organization by body part listed here, (2) use the following Anatomical Contents pages to find the appropriate pages, (3) use the section labels at the top of pages, or (4) use the index at the end of this book.

The forty specific treatment plans in Part III are organized by body parts in roughly a head-to-toe manner, as follows:

CONDITION	PAGE
1. Neck—Herniated disk	47
2. Chest—Fracture of the vertebra and rib	51
3. Back—Herniated or slipped disk	54
4. Back—Muscle tear	58
5. Shoulder—Acromioclavicular joint (AC) separation	61
6. Shoulder—Anterior dislocation	65
7. Shoulder—Rotator cuff tendinitis and tear	69
8. Shoulder—Rupture of biceps tendon	73
9. Shoulder—Subacromial bursitis	76
10. Elbow—Lateral epicondylitis (tennis elbow)	79
11. Elbow—Medial epicondylitis (baseball elbow)	82
12. Elbow—Ulnar nerve entrapment	85

CONDITION	PAGE
13. Wrist—Carpal tunnel	88
14. Wrist—Scaphoid bone fracture (navicular bone)	91
15. Wrist—Ulnar neuritis (biker's wrist)	94
16. Finger—Extensor tendon tear (baseball finger)	97
17. Finger—Ruptured ulnar collateral ligament (skier's thumb)	100
18. Hip—Tear of adductor muscles (inner thigh)	103
19. Hip—Stress fracture of the neck of the femur	107
20. Hip—Trochanteric bursitis	111
21. Thigh—Myositis ossificans, heterotopic bone formation	114
22. Thigh—Quadriceps muscle tear	117
23. Thigh—Hamstring muscle tear	120
24. Knee—Anterior cruciate ligament (ACL) tear	123
25. Knee—Chondromalacia patella	127
26. Knee—Iliotibial band syndrome	131
27. Knee—Osgood-Schlatter disease	134
28. Knee—Osteoarthritis	137
29. Knee—Kneecap (patella) dislocation	141
30. Knee—Patellar tendinitis (jumper's knee)	145
31. Knee—Torn meniscus	148
32. Shin—Shin splints	151
33. Shin—Tibia or fibula stress fracture	154
34. Calf—Rupture of the gastrocnemius muscle	157
35. Ankle—Achilles tendinitis	161
36. Ankle—Torn Achilles tendon	164
37. Ankle—Lateral ligament sprain	167
38. Foot—Metatarsal stress fracture	170
39. Foot—Morton's neuroma	173
40. Foot—Plantar fasciitis (heel pain)	176

Each condition presents a specific 6-Point Condition Summary and a specific 10-Point Treatment Plan (see Part II for a general description). With this information, you can learn to listen to your body and establish the best activity level for your outdoor recreational injury. All advice in Part III can be used after you have had a correct diagnosis of your problem from a health care professional. The specific rehabilitation exercise programs mentioned in each 10-Point Treatment Plan can be found in Part IV.

Anatomical Contents

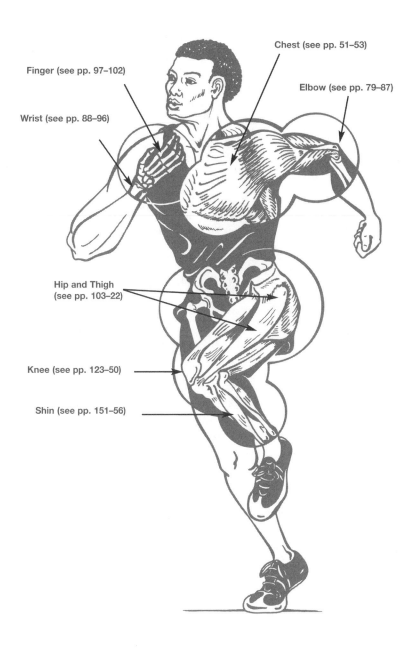

Chest (see pp. 51–53)

Elbow (see pp. 79–87)

Finger (see pp. 97–102)

Wrist (see pp. 88–96)

Hip and Thigh
(see pp. 103–22)

Knee (see pp. 123–50)

Shin (see pp. 151–56)

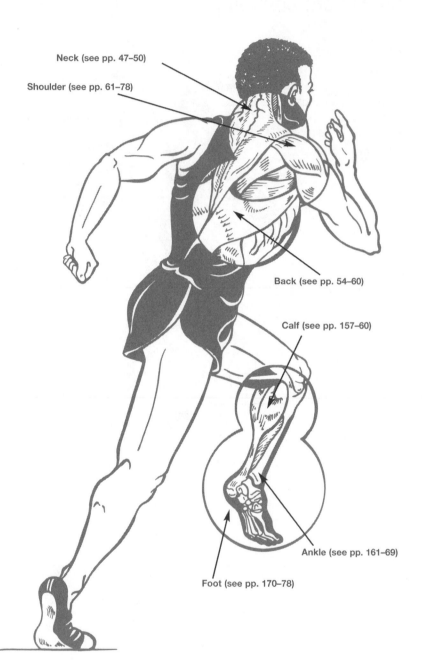

Neck (see pp. 47–50)

Shoulder (see pp. 61–78)

Back (see pp. 54–60)

Calf (see pp. 157–60)

Ankle (see pp. 161–69)

Foot (see pp. 170–78)

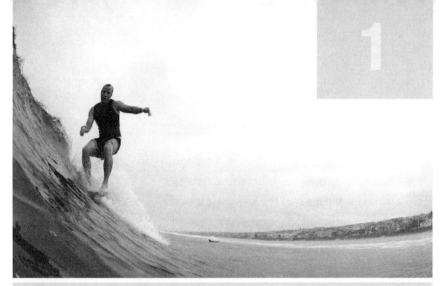

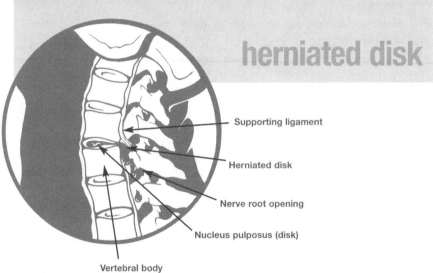

herniated disk

Supporting ligament

Herniated disk

Nerve root opening

Nucleus pulposus (disk)

Vertebral body

6-POINT CONDITION STATEMENT

1. Definition

A mechanical condition characterized by intense pain in the neck radiating down the arm, caused by nerve irritation from a disk degeneration, herniation, or bone spur.

2. Cause

- Acute local trauma to the neck from intense twisting in activities such as surfing or skiing.
- Chronic excessive twisting and hyperextension of the neck, causing undue pressure on the cervical disk and nerve root.

3. Subjective Symptoms

- Pain radiates from the back and side of the neck down to the shoulder, arm, and hand.
- Numbness or tingling radiates down the arm.
- Local swelling generally is not perceived.
- Stiffness in the neck exists, especially with extension and rotation.
- Sneezing and coughing aggravate the pain and radiation.

4. Objective Findings

- Motion of the neck is very restricted, especially in hyperextension and twisting.
- Motor and sensory deficits may exist in the arm, with reduced sensation and strength.
- Compression of the head and neck aggravates the pain.

5. Testing Procedures

- Routine x-rays can be normal but will usually show straightening of the normal cervical curvature. Narrowing and spur formation around the nerve root and disks are usually present.
- MRI tests may show disk herniation.
- A CAT scan may be helpful.

6. Prognosis

As with most nerve injuries, healing is very prolonged. Any impact, twisting, and extension maneuvers should be removed from outdoor recreational activity. If pain persists, hospitalization and traction may be necessary. Some patients need surgery to remove the disks and possibly fuse the spine for extreme degeneration.

10-POINT TREATMENT PLAN

1. Activity Levels

- During periods of pain, avoid impact activities such as running.
- Walking, swimming, and biking may be satisfactory.

- If pain is caused by twisting of the neck while swimming, use a snorkel to breathe with the neck straight.

2. Alternative Exercises

- Walking, swimming, and biking are excellent straight activities.
- As pain subsides, return to light twisting activities. Avoid impact.
- Use a mountain bicycle for biking so that you do not have to bend over and hyperextend the neck.
- Use a walking/trekking stick to reduce stress on the joint.

3. Rehab Exercises

- See rehabilitation exercise program in Part IV of this book.
- Do isometric exercises with local hand pressure to maintain muscle tone without moving the neck. As pain subsides, gradually increase motion and strength.

4. Support

- Use a simple wrap (like a towel) around the neck if a collar is not available. A semirigid collar may be of help during walking, running, and biking.

5. Thermal Treatment

- Use local heat to reduce muscle spasm.
- Local pain can be treated with ice massage.

6. Medication

- For oral medication see "The 10-Point Treatment Plan" in Part II of this book.
- Avoid strong narcotics because of the chronic nature of the problem.
- Trigger point injections (at the site of muscle spasm) with steroid and Xylocaine sometimes help.

7. Equipment

- Use a hyperextension pad, such as in football equipment, to prevent the neck and head from overextending.

8. Nutrition

- Avoid weight gain during periods of inactivity.
- See nutrition suggestions in Part V of this book.

9. Fluids

- Maintain excellent hydration.

10. Surfaces

- Avoid jarring on hard surfaces such as hard roads and concrete.

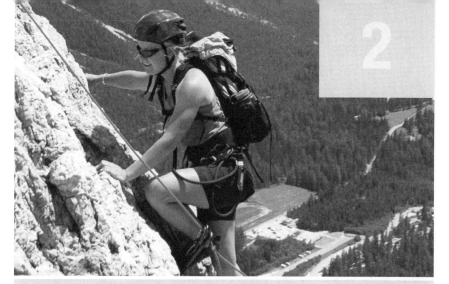

fracture of the vertebra and rib

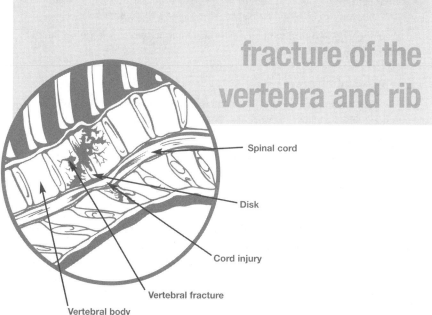

Spinal cord

Disk

Cord injury

Vertebral fracture

Vertebral body

6-POINT CONDITION STATEMENT

1. Definition

A traumatic condition associated with direct trauma to the bone of the thoracic vertebra or the adjacent rib structure.

2. Cause

- Compression (such as falling from a height) or a sudden jarring (such as bouncing in a toboggan) can cause thoracic spine injury.

- Rib fractures can occur from direct impact from rock and mountain climbing or falling in skiing.

3. Subjective Symptoms

- Well-localized pain exists at the bony site.
- Local swelling may be present from the hematoma (collection of blood).
- Local stiffness occurs from spasm of the adjacent muscles.

4. Objective Findings

- Coughing and sneezing are very painful.
- Nerve symptoms, such as radiating pain and numbness, may occur in the leg if the fracture is very severe and compresses the spinal cord.
- Coughing of blood and difficulty with breathing may occur if the rib injury seriously injures the lung.

5. Testing Procedures

- Routine x-ray is very important for the rib, the lung, and the bone of the thoracic spine to find a bone injury or fluid in the lung.
- Initial x-rays could be negative if the fracture is minimal.
- Bone scan and MRI may be helpful in the first few days to pinpoint the fracture.

6. Prognosis

With no displacement of the fracture, healing is slow but progressive, with excellent results. Some thoracic fractures, if displaced, may require stabilization surgery, especially if there is spinal cord involvement. Rib fractures generally heal with minimal immobilization. In rare cases, a rib fracture is serious and could puncture the lung and require immediate pulmonary management.

10-POINT TREATMENT PLAN

1. Activity Levels

- Rest is initial activity, followed gradually by deep breathing, coughing, and gentle thoracic exercises during the first week.

2. Alternative Exercises

- Nonimpact exercises are helpful—simple walking, swimming, and biking.

- Gradually progress within a week or two to light stationary biking, followed by outdoor biking, depending on the type of fracture.
- Light jogging can be considered if there is no pain at 6 to 12 weeks. Let pain be the guide.

3. Rehab Exercises

- See rehabilitation exercise program in Part IV of this book.
- Rest is the treatment for the first several weeks.
- Gradually start deep breathing and mobilization exercises of the thoracic musculature.
- Begin simple push-ups and partial sit-ups as pain subsides.

4. Support

- A rib belt is very helpful.
- If the thoracic fracture is extensive, a fabricated metal or plastic hyperextension brace may be indicated.

5. Thermal Treatment

- Local ice to reduce swelling.
- Gradual use of heat to reduce muscle spasm.

6. Medication

- For oral medication, see "The 10-Point Treatment Plan" in Part II of this book.

7. Equipment

- A rib belt or a 6-inch elastic bandage wrapped around the thoracic spine is very helpful initially.
- More rigid thoracic supports may be in order if the fracture is severe.
- Use a trekking/walking stick to reduce stress on the joint.

8. Nutrition

- Avoid weight gain during periods of inactivity.
- See nutrition suggestions in Part V of this book.

9. Fluids

- Maintain excellent hydration.

10. Surfaces

- Sleeping on a very firm mattress to control the spine is quite important. Training should be done on soft surfaces to avoid jarring.

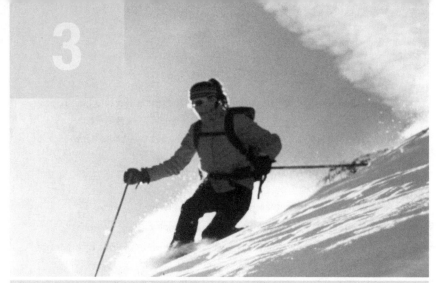

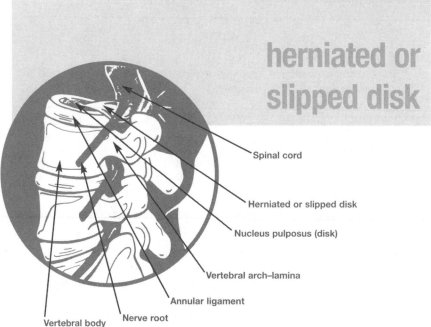

herniated or slipped disk

Spinal cord

Herniated or slipped disk

Nucleus pulposus (disk)

Vertebral arch–lamina

Annular ligament

Nerve root

Vertebral body

6-POINT CONDITION STATEMENT

1. Definition

A traumatic or degenerative condition characterized by localized breakdown or slipping of the nucleus pulposus (lumbar disk), causing direct inflammation and pressure on the lumbar nerve.

2. Cause

- Sudden exertion or extreme twisting, such as in skiing, especially with the back in an extended position, causes a tear of the ligaments around the disk. This results in pressure and inflammation around the nerve root, lead-ing to intense pain radiating down the back of the leg (sciatica).

- In a middle-aged athlete (around age 40), the tissues are starting to wear. A sudden twisting maneuver causes breakdown of the connective tissue, leading to direct inflammation of the nerve.

3. Subjective Symptoms

- Acute, sharp pain in the lumbar spine radiating into the hip and down to the leg.
- Numbness and tingling down the leg, aggravated by strain, such as cough-ing or sitting.
- Muscles guarded (tight) and spasmodic, especially with lumbar positions in extension.
- Pain aggravated by long periods of sitting, such as while driving a car; pain relieved with standing.
- Sneezing and coughing are very painful.

4. Objective Findings

- Back motion is very guarded, especially with extension.
- Lumbar stability is good.
- Straight-leg raising is very painful, with radiation of the pain from the back down the leg.
- Neurologic testing may reveal loss of sensation, reduced muscle power, and reduced reflexes.

5. Testing Procedures

- Initial x-rays may be normal or may show early signs of wearing and thin-ning of the lumbar disk spaces.
- An MRI test may be positive and may show a herniated disk.
- A CAT scan may be positive and may show a lumbar disk herniation.
- EMG nerve testing after several weeks may show the nerve injury.

6. Prognosis

Healing can be very slow because of the nerve injury. Referral to a pain spe-cialist for possible epidural injections may be required if rest at home does not help after 1 or 2 weeks. Surgery may be necessary if pain persists or increasing neurologic deficits develop after several weeks.

10-POINT TREATMENT PLAN

1. Activity Levels

- Avoid any exercise that includes impact, twisting, or bending; err on the side of overresting.
- As pain subsides, start to walk, then swim, and then bike.
- Avoid activities that include impact for at least 6 weeks.

2. Alternative Exercises

- Use a stationary bicycle and swim during the initial weeks of rehabilitation.
- Avoid anything that will hyperextend and twist the spine.
- Run in a swimming pool.

3. Rehab Exercises

- See rehabilitation exercise program in Part IV of this book.
- Rest is indicated, especially with the knees bent.
- Deep breathing and gentle leg and arm motion are helpful during early periods of pain.
- During periods of rehabilitation, do sit-ups and flexion exercises to maintain abdominal strength.

4. Support

- A lumbar brace can be tried but should not be a substitute for good judgment—let pain be the guide.

5. Thermal Treatment

- Because of the muscle spasm, initial heat is best for muscle relaxation.
- Heat is more effective for large muscle groups. Switch to ice when the pain becomes localized.

6. Medication

- For oral medication, see "The 10-Point Treatment Plan" in Part II of this book.

7. Equipment

- Lie on a very firm surface, such as the floor or a very firm mattress.

8. Nutrition

- Avoid weight gain during periods of inactivity.
- See nutrition suggestions in Part V of this book.
- Because of bed rest, avoid overeating.
- Don't overeat during periods of frustration and depression.

9. Fluids

- Maintain excellent hydration.

10. Surfaces

- Avoid hills and hard surfaces during rehabilitation.
- Stay on blacktop and bicycle paths for exercise.
- Sleep on very firm surfaces.

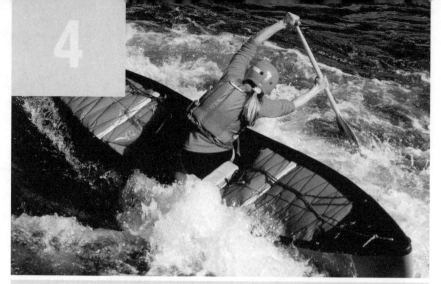

muscle tear

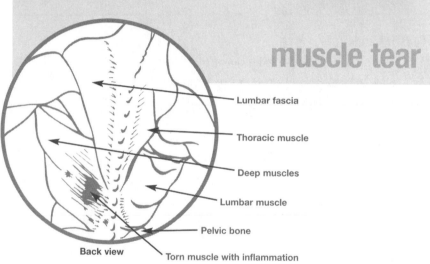

Lumbar fascia

Thoracic muscle

Deep muscles

Lumbar muscle

Pelvic bone

Back view

Torn muscle with inflammation

6-POINT CONDITION STATEMENT

1. Definition

A traumatic condition characterized by a local tearing of the muscle of the lower back, causing local pain, spasm, and occasional radiation of discomfort.

2. Cause

- Localized muscle tearing due to a rapid twisting maneuver, generally with the spine in either extreme flexion or extension.
- Injuries such as bruising from direct impact, such as in paddling or canoeing.

3. Subjective Symptoms

- Well-localized pain in the lower back area with occasional radiation to the hip and groin.
- Tightness of muscle, especially with bending; pain aggravated by sneezing, coughing, and sitting.
- Neurologic symptoms such as numbness or intense radiation down the leg generally not present.

4. Objective Findings

- Motion of the lumbar spine is restricted, especially in flexion or tension.
- Stability of the spine is good.
- Muscles are generally tight, but there is no swelling. Neurologic exam is negative.

5. Testing Procedures

- Routine x-rays are generally normal.
- Neurologic exam and special nerve tests are negative.
- MRI is generally not helpful, unless severe soft-tissue muscle injury is present.

6. Prognosis

Healing potential is good but can be very prolonged, taking weeks to months. Some cases require bed rest if the muscle injury is serious. Surgery is not indicated, unless a herniated disk is associated.

10-POINT TREATMENT PLAN

1. Activity Levels

- Keep knees bent during the period of rest (on a bed or a semireclining chair).
- Straight activities such as walking, swimming, and biking are best at the beginning of recovery.

2. Alternative Exercises

- Use a trekking/walking stick to reduce stress on the joint.
- Use a stationary bicycle and swim during the initial weeks of rehabilitation.
- Avoid anything that will hyperextend and twist the spine.
- Run in a swimming pool.

3. Rehab Exercises

- See rehabilitation exercise program in Part IV of this book.
- First, rest in bed, keeping the knees bent.
- As pain subsides, within a few days to a week, begin gentle flexion and extension exercises such as sit-ups, push-ups, and swimming.

4. Support

- Various lumbar supports are available.
- Wrap several elastic bandages around the lumbar spine.
- Initially, taping can be used.
- Lumbar corsets are available to help protect the spine during early return to activities.

5. Thermal Treatment

- Use local ice massage to reduce spasm.
- If large muscle groups are involved, heat can be tried before ice for muscle relaxation.

6. Medication

- For oral medication, see "The 10-Point Treatment Plan" in Part II of this book.
- Muscle relaxers may be prescribed. (*Note:* May cause sleepiness.)
- Sometimes a local steroid injection may be indicated in the inflamed muscle after weeks of rehabilitation.

7. Equipment

- Wrap the lumbar spine with elastic bandages or corset to protect the back.

8. Nutrition

- Avoid weight gain during periods of inactivity.
- See nutrition suggestions in Part V of this book.

9. Fluids

- Maintain excellent hydration.

10. Surfaces

- Avoid hills, which will aggravate the lumbar strain.
- Use flat, soft surfaces such as blacktops and bicycle paths for early exercise routines.
- Sleep on very firm surfaces.

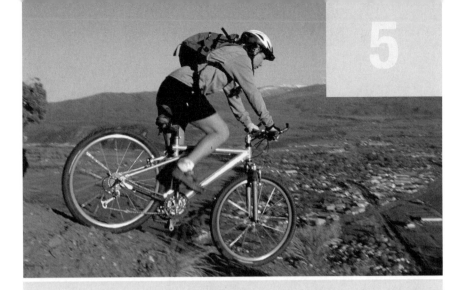

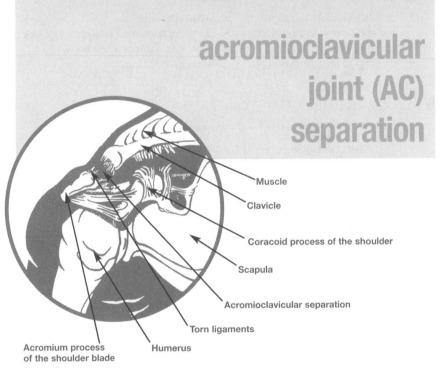

acromioclavicular joint (AC) separation

- Muscle
- Clavicle
- Coracoid process of the shoulder
- Scapula
- Acromioclavicular separation
- Torn ligaments
- Acromium process of the shoulder blade
- Humerus

6-POINT CONDITION STATEMENT

1. Definition

A traumatic displacement and separation at the end of the collar bone (clavicle) from the tip of the shoulder (acromion) due to violent tearing of the ligaments that stabilize the clavicle. There are three grades:

Grade I—Minimal displacement
Grade II—Moderate displacement
Grade III—Severe displacement (may require surgery)

2. Cause

- Direct fall on the side of the shoulder, as during rock climbing or mountain climbing.
- Indirect fall on an outstretched arm, causing the clavicle to displace due to torn ligaments, as during skiing.

3. Subjective Symptoms

Acute

- Sudden pain at the top of the shoulder following a fall
- Local swelling
- Inability to lift arm overhead

Chronic

- Ache with use
- Grinding sensation with shoulder use
- Pain with overhead activities such as throwing

4. Objective Findings

Acute

- Well-localized tenderness at the tip of the clavicle at the AC joint.
- Local swelling.
- Local deformity
- Negative neurovascular test
- Shoulder motion restricted

Chronic

- A small spur or bump may be palpated at the AC joint.
- Local swelling may be present.
- Crepitation or noise can be heard or felt
- Motion is almost normal but may be restricted on extreme overhead motion

5. Testing Procedures

- Routine x-rays vary, revealing minimal displacement in Grade I to extreme displacement in Grade III.
- Bone scan may be positive for bone inflammation in chronic cases.
- MRI test may be helpful for showing tear of the ligaments and meniscus of the joint.

6. Prognosis

Healing is generally very satisfactory in Grade I and Grade II cases. Grade III cases may be left with a painful bump and deformity on the tip of the shoulder. In most cases, this bump and deformity do not limit function but may be associated with moderate weakness. Some surgeons will recommend surgical repair in Grade III cases to restore the anatomy in high-performance athletes.

10-POINT TREATMENT PLAN

1. Activity Levels

- Immobilization of the shoulder with a sling for Grade I and Grade II tears. Grade III tears may require surgery or a special harness.

2. Alternative Exercises

- May walk, lightly jog, and bike.
- Running in a swimming pool is permitted, but arm motion is not.
- Use a trekking/walking stick to reduce stress on the joint when shoulder pain subsides.

3. Rehab Exercises

- See rehabilitation exercise program in Part IV of this book.
- Do isometric tightening exercises to maintain muscle tone during initial period of immobilization and sling.
- Gradually increase muscle flexibility, endurance, speed, and strength with gentle weight lifting as the sling becomes unnecessary.

4. Support

- First aid consists of a sling and elastic wraps.
- Special harness for acromioclavicular joint in selected cases.

5. Thermal Treatment

- Local ice to reduce pain and inflammation for the first 1 or 2 days.
- Local heat to reduce muscle spasm after the first few days.

6. Medication

- For oral medication, see "The 10-Point Treatment Plan" in Part II of this book.
- After several months of local pain and inflammation, a local steroid injection may be indicated.

7. Equipment

- During periods of immobilization, leg exercises and biking are permissible.

8. Nutrition

- Avoid weight gain during periods of inactivity.
- See nutrition suggestions in Part V of this book.

9. Fluids

- Maintain excellent hydration.

10. Surfaces

- Use nonskid running surfaces to avoid falls on the arm.

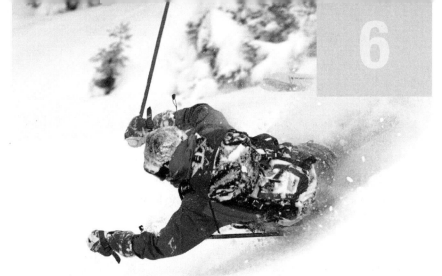

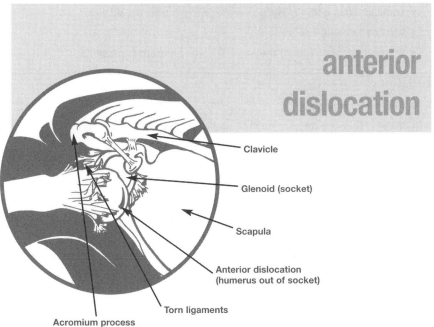

Clavicle

Glenoid (socket)

Scapula

Anterior dislocation
(humerus out of socket)

Torn ligaments

Acromium process

6-POINT CONDITION STATEMENT

1. Definition

A traumatic condition in which the ball of the shoulder (humerus) completely sep-
arates from a socket (glenoid). The displacement is usually forward (anterior).

2. Cause

- In outdoor recreation, this would occur in traumatic falls such as mountain climbing or downhill skiing.
- Direct trauma to the side of the shoulder during a fall on the shoulder.
- Indirect shoulder trauma by fall on the outstretched hand.
- Congenital looseness (laxity) of the joint due to bony abnormality or ligament insufficiency.

3. Subjective Symptoms

- Acute, intense pain on the front of the shoulder.
- Local swelling and a mass perceived (the humerus bone).
- Inability to move the arm.
- Occasional numbness in the hand, if nerve pressure is present.

4. Objective Findings

- Arm rotated outward.
- Inability to move the arm due to pain, weakness, and deformity.
- Bony mass felt on the front of the shoulder.
- Nerve exam usually normal, but nerve damage present in some cases.

5. Testing Procedures

- X-ray will show displacement of the head of the humerus. Associated fracture may be present.
- Bone scan and MRI are not needed in early cases but may be helpful in chronic recurrent cases.

6. Prognosis

Most cases heal if proper rest and immobilization are done in acute cases. Teenage patients have a higher rate of recurrence. Immediate closed reduction (putting the shoulder back in place) after an x-ray is required. Often this is done with a local or general anesthetic. Some cases develop recurrent dislocation, which may require surgical stabilization. Certain rotation motions may have to be avoided. The return to outdoor recreational activities is often delayed several months until flexibility, endurance, speed, and strength are improved.

10-POINT TREATMENT PLAN

1. Activity Levels

- Complete immobilization of the shoulder for several weeks to allow healing of the injured muscles and ligaments.
- Begin a gradual program of pendulum swinging of the arm, leading to full-motion exercises.

2. Alternative Activities

- Walking, stationary biking, and light jogging are permitted if pain is minimal and there is no jarring.

3. Rehab Exercises

- See rehabilitation exercise program in Part IV of this book.
- During sling immobilization of the first month, do isometric tightening of the shoulder and neck muscles.
- Once sling is removed, start exercises to build flexibility, endurance, speed, and strength by using tubing and free weights.

4. Support

- Acute phase: first aid in a sling or wrapping the shoulder with an elastic bandage.
- Post reduction: sling and shoulder wrap.
- Rehabilitation: simple collar and cuff to allow pendulum exercises and gradual mobilization.

5. Thermal Treatment

- Local ice to the shoulder for the first 1 or 2 days to reduce pain and swelling.
- Local heat to reduce muscle spasm after 1 or 2 days.

6. Medication

- For oral medication, see "The 10-Point Treatment Plan" in Part II of this book.
- Acute pain is treated with codeine and possibly a narcotic injection for the closed reduction.

- A local steroid injection sometimes is required for scarring and inflammation several months after rehabilitation.

7. Equipment

- A special shoulder harness may be used for outdoor recreation to prevent external rotation and recurrent dislocation.

8. Nutrition

- Avoid weight gain during periods of inactivity.
- See nutrition suggestions in Part V of this book.

9. Fluids

- Maintain excellent hydration.
- Immediately after the injury avoid drinking because of the possibility of needing closed reduction under general anesthesia.

10. Surfaces

- Light running and twisting activities may be done on nonskid surfaces to prevent slipping and reinjuring the arm.

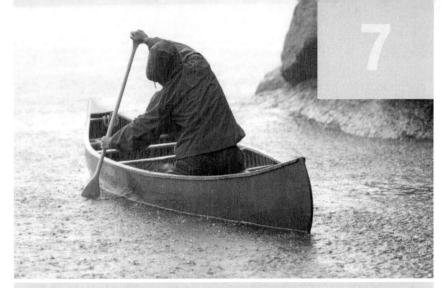

rotator cuff tendinitis and tear

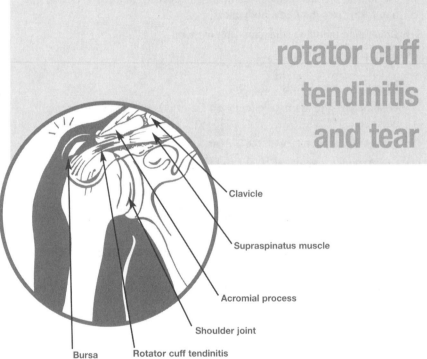

Clavicle

Supraspinatus muscle

Acromial process

Shoulder joint

Bursa   Rotator cuff tendinitis

6-POINT CONDITION STATEMENT

1. Definition

A local overuse inflammation to the group of four major shoulder muscles that run together, attach to the humerus, and form a heavy tendon called the rotator cuff. Overhead activities may impinge the cuff and cause wear and tear.

2. Cause

- Repeated shoulder activities such as in canoeing or kayaking will stretch and impinge the cuff, causing local wear and tear.
- Acute symptoms may occur in a sudden fall.

3. Subjective Symptoms

- Pain well localized to the anterior lateral aspect of the shoulder just below the acromion. The symptoms may radiate around the shoulder or down the arm.
- Stiffness and difficulty with overhead activities.
- Weakness, a common major complaint, especially difficulty in pulling the arm away from the body (abduction).
- Crepitation (grinding sensation with motion).
- Night pain is common.

4. Objective Findings

- Well-localized tenderness directly on the rotator cuff at the tip of the acromion.
- Weakness, especially with the arm at 90 degrees.
- Crepitation is sometimes heard and felt.

5. Testing Procedures

- Regular x-rays generally are negative, but chronic cases may show calcification or spurs.
- A bone scan is generally not diagnostic but may show inflammation of the bone.
- An arthrogram can be very helpful in large incomplete and complete tears.
- MRI studies show early signs of wearing.

6. Prognosis

The healing potential is not excellent because of the poor blood supply. Restrict activities that cause the condition. If symptoms persist, surgery in the form of arthroscopy or major open procedures may be necessary to debride and repair the tendon.

10-POINT TREATMENT PLAN

1. Activity Levels

- Restrict extreme overhead activities.
- Modify throwing and outdoor recreational activities to keep the shoulder below 90 degrees.

2. Alternative Exercises

- Avoid twisting and torqueing activities.
- Work more on biking, swimming, and running.
- Gradually increase shoulder activities in a moderate program.

3. Rehab Exercises

- See rehabilitation exercise program in Part IV of this book.
- Progressive stiffness must be prevented.
- Flexibility and strengthening exercises are very important.

4. Support

- Braces are generally not effective, but gentle wrapping of the shoulder with an elastic wrap sometimes will help during acute pain.

5. Thermal Treatment

- Local ice to reduce inflammation of the surrounding tendon and bursa
- Local heat to relax and mobilize the tight shoulder muscles

6. Medication

- For oral medication, see "The 10-Point Treatment Plan" in Part II of this book.
- Progress to local steroid injection before considering surgery.

7. Equipment

- Proper selection of paddling and kayaking equipment to prevent shoulder stress is very important.
- Choose equipment that has minimal vibration.

8. Nutrition

- Avoid weight gain during periods of inactivity.
- See nutrition suggestions in Part V of this book.

9. Fluids

- Maintain excellent hydration.

10. Surfaces

- Minimize jarring by avoiding running on concrete and excessively banked or curved hills.

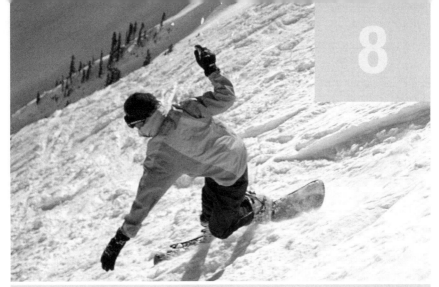

rupture of biceps tendon

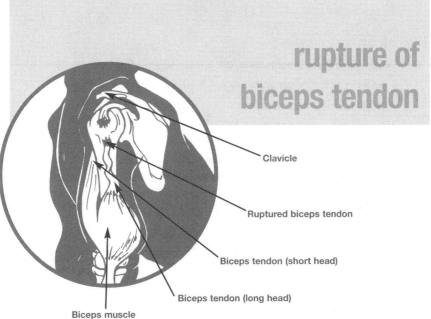

Clavicle

Ruptured biceps tendon

Biceps tendon (short head)

Biceps tendon (long head)

Biceps muscle

6-POINT CONDITION STATEMENT

1. Definition

A traumatic overuse condition resulting in a sudden tearing of the biceps tendon in the front of the shoulder.

2. Cause

- Violent, heavy lifting that overloads the tendon, resulting in tearing.
- Repetitive, overhead lifting, generally in a middle-aged person.

3. Subjective Symptoms

- Acute pain and perception of a "pop" on the front of the shoulder.
- Sudden weakness with lifting.
- Muscle mass perceived and felt in the front of the mid-arm.

4. Objective Findings

- Local tenderness directly on the front of the shoulder, 2 to 3 inches below the clavicle.
- Local swelling possible with bruising.
- Weakness of flexor muscle group.
- Nerve function test.

5. Testing Procedures

- X-rays generally are not helpful, but a spur may be present.
- Bone scan and MRI generally are not required to make the diagnosis.
- Arthroscopy is rarely indicated.

6. Prognosis

Surgery is rarely indicated. Weakness is rarely a problem after adequate rehabilitation. Healing is usually accomplished without surgery.

10-POINT TREATMENT PLAN

1. Activity Levels

- Let pain be the guide for the first month.
- No lifting is allowed during the first month, but isometric exercises are permitted to maintain muscle tone.

2. Alternative Exercises

- Running, biking, swimming, and running in a swimming pool are all permitted.

3. Rehab Exercises

- See rehabilitation exercise program in Part IV of this book.
- Light flexion exercises during the acute phase.
- Shoulder rehabilitation exercises with tubing and sandbags.

4. Support

- Sling for 1 to 2 weeks.

5. Thermal Treatment

- Local ice for the initial 1 or 2 days for pain and swelling.
- Local heat after a few days for muscle spasm.

6. Medication

- For oral medication, see "The 10-Point Treatment Plan" in Part II of this book.
- If chronic pain persists after several months, a local steroid injection may be indicated.

7. Equipment

- Modification of intense weight-lifting equipment to simple free weights.

8. Nutrition

- Avoid weight gain during periods of inactivity.
- See nutrition suggestions in Part V of this book.

9. Fluids

- Maintain excellent hydration.

10. Surfaces

- A nonskid surface should be used to avoid any further falls on an out-stretched arm.

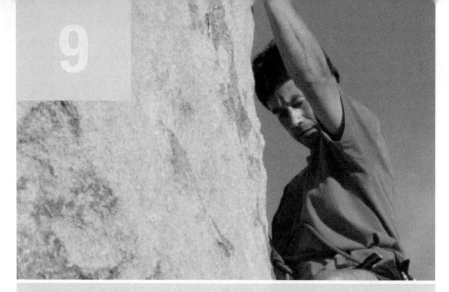

subacromial bursitis

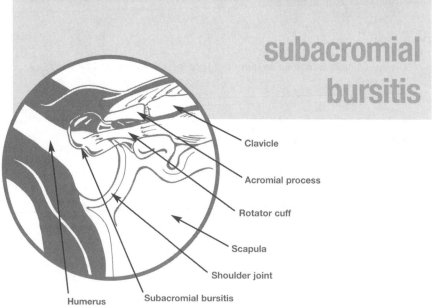

Clavicle

Acromial process

Rotator cuff

Scapula

Shoulder joint

Humerus   Subacromial bursitis

6-POINT CONDITION STATEMENT

1. Definition

A traumatic overuse condition characterized by local pain and stiffness due to inflammation in the bursa and tendon between the bones of the shoulder.

2. Cause

- Repetitive overhead arm use, such as in rock climbing.
- Direct trauma or fall on the side of the shoulder.
- Early tear of the rotator cuff, resulting in inflammation of the bursa.

3. Subjective Symptoms

- Pain with shoulder use, usually overhead.
- Noise and crepitation with shoulder use.
- Swelling usually not present.
- Stiffness is moderate.

4. Objective Findings

- Tenderness is well localized to the tip of the shoulder just below the point of the shoulder (acromion).
- Swelling is usually not perceived by the physician.
- There is pain, along with limitation of arm movement away from the body (abduction).

5. Testing Procedures

- X-ray is usually negative in early cases. Late cases may show local spurring and degenerative changes.
- Scan may show bone inflammation.
- Arthrogram may show small tears in the tendon.
- MRI may be helpful, showing the early signs of wearing.
- Arthroscopy in chronic cases may show inflammation of the bursa and tendon.

6. Prognosis

With rest and restriction of activity, pain and inflammation usually subside. Some cases require more aggressive treatment with anti-inflammatory medication, steroid injection, and possibly arthroscopic shaving and removal of the bursa.

10-POINT TREATMENT PLAN

1. Activity Levels

- Let pain be the guide.
- Minimize overhead activities.

2. Alternative Exercises

- Running, biking, and swimming are permitted.
- Hiking without rock climbing is permitted.

3. Rehab Exercises

- See rehabilitation exercise program in Part IV of this book.
- Use gentle pendulum range of motion to loosen the shoulder, and progressively use tubing and sandbags to maintain flexibility, endurance, speed, and strength.

4. Support

- Braces and slings are generally not helpful.

5. Thermal Treatment

- Local ice massage after pain or after exercise workout.
- Heat before activity to relax muscles.

6. Medication

- For oral medication, see "The 10-Point Treatment Plan" in Part II of this book.
- Local steroid injection is sometimes very helpful.

7. Equipment

- Isokinetic exercises for the upper shoulder to maintain shoulder strength.
- Aerodyne bicycle for arm and leg use.

8. Nutrition

- Avoid weight gain during periods of inactivity.
- See nutrition suggestions in Part V of this book.

9. Fluids

- Maintain excellent hydration.

10. Surfaces

- Hike or climb on nonskid surfaces to avoid falling on outstretched arm.

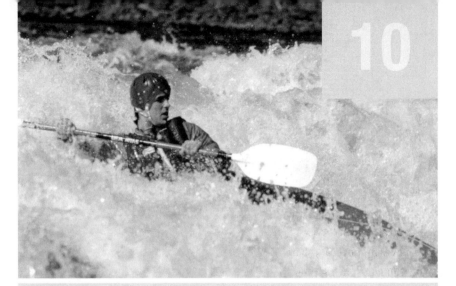

lateral epicondylitis (tennis elbow)

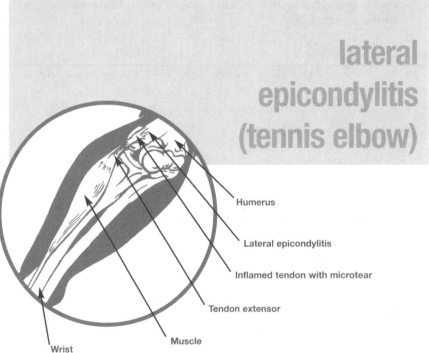

Humerus

Lateral epicondylitis

Inflamed tendon with microtear

Tendon extensor

Muscle

Wrist

6-POINT CONDITION STATEMENT

1. Definition

A local inflammation on the outer (lateral) side of the elbow at the lateral epicondyle, due to repeated microtrauma, resulting in local elbow pain.

2. Cause

- Acute, sudden, violent injury and tearing of the muscle.
- Chronic, repeated strain and pulling of the extensor forearm muscles with repeated paddling activities.

3. Subjective Symptoms

- Pain is well localized to the outer (lateral) side of the elbow. The pain may radiate down the forearm.
- Swelling generally is not present.
- Stiffness may be present but generally is not a feature.
- Pain is aggravated by wrist activities such as lifting a heavy object with the palm down (pronated).

4. Objective Findings

- Tenderness well localized to the muscle attachment to the side of the elbow.
- Weakness of the wrist extensor group due to pain and inflammation.
- Loss of motion is not present.

5. Testing Procedures

- Routine x-rays generally are negative, but a small spur may be present in the elbow.
- Bone scan may be of help in showing local inflammation.
- EMG studies are usually negative.
- MRI studies generally are not helpful.

6. Prognosis

Healing in the tendon can be prolonged because of poor blood supply to the tendon. After months of conservative treatment for inflammation, surgery may be necessary to remove the offending scar tissue.

10-POINT TREATMENT PLAN

1. Activity Levels

- Continue moderate paddling activities in quiet water.

2. Alternative Exercises

- Running, biking, and swimming are very helpful for maintaining aerobic exercise.

3. Rehab Exercises

- See rehabilitation exercise program in Part IV of this book.
- Maintain a balance of exercises to develop flexibility and strength, especially in the wrist extensor group.

4. Support

- A tennis elbow band, worn 1 to 2 inches below the elbow, helps compress and immobilize the muscle group.

5. Thermal Treatment

- Local ice massage is very helpful.
- Use heat to mobilize muscles.

6. Medication

- For oral medication, see "The 10-Point Treatment Plan" in Part II of this book.

7. Equipment

- Choose equipment that has thick hand grips.

8. Nutrition

- Avoid weight gain during periods of inactivity.
- See nutrition suggestions in Part V of this book.

9. Fluids

- Maintain excellent hydration.

10. Surfaces

- Run on bike paths (asphalt is best). Avoid running on concrete, which will further jar the body.

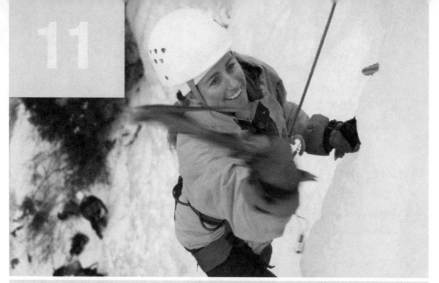

medial epicondylitis (baseball elbow)

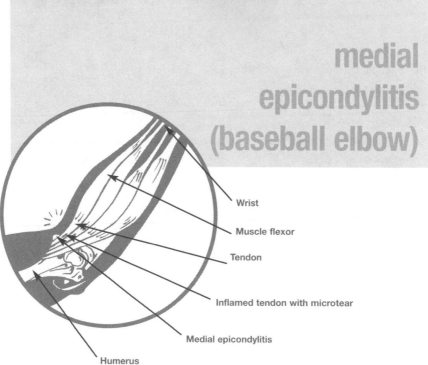

Wrist

Muscle flexor

Tendon

Inflamed tendon with microtear

Medial epicondylitis

Humerus

6-POINT CONDITION STATEMENT

1. Definition

A local traumatic condition on the inner (medial) aspect of the elbow at the medial epicondyle, due to repetitive microtrauma or twisting.

2. Cause

- Acute, sudden throwing injury due to violent twisting of the elbow.
- Chronic repetitive strain and pulling of the flexor forearm muscles during climbing activities.

3. Subjective Symptoms

- Pain well localized at the inner aspect of the elbow, with pain radiating to the inner forearm.
- Swelling generally is not present.
- Stiffness may be present but generally is not a feature.
- Pain aggravated by lifting objects with the palm up (supinated).
- Numbness is not a feature, unless there is ulnar nerve involvement.

4. Objective Findings

- Tenderness well localized at the muscle attachment to the inner side of the elbow.
- Weakness in forearm flexion of the wrist.
- Motion generally intact.
- Nerve exam negative.

5. Testing Procedures

- Routine x-rays generally are negative, but a small spur may be present on the medial elbow.
- EMG studies generally are negative.
- MRI studies usually are not helpful.

6. Prognosis

Healing of the tendon may be prolonged because of poor blood supply at the muscle–tendon junction. After months of conservative treatment for inflammation, surgery may be necessary to remove offending scar tissue and bone spurs.

10-POINT TREATMENT PLAN

1. Activity Levels

- Continue to participate in moderate hiking and rock climbing, but avoid excessive forearm maneuvers.

2. Alternative Exercises

- Running, biking, and swimming are all very helpful for maintaining aerobic exercise.

3. Rehab Exercises

- See rehabilitation exercise program in Part IV of this book.
- Maintain a balance of exercises to develop flexibility and strength, especially in the wrist flexor muscle group.

4. Support

- A tennis elbow band is not as helpful as it is on the lateral side of the elbow.

5. Thermal Treatment

- Local ice massage is very helpful in reducing inflammation.
- Use heat to mobilize muscles before activity.

6. Medication

- For oral medication, see "The 10-Point Treatment Plan" in Part II of this book.
- Progress to local steroid injection before considering surgery.

7. Equipment

- Chose equipment that has thick hand grips.

8. Nutrition

- Avoid weight gain during periods of inactivity.
- See nutrition suggestions in Part V of this book.

9. Fluids

- Maintain excellent hydration.

10. Surfaces

- Run on bike paths (asphalt is best). Avoid running on concrete, which may further jar the body.

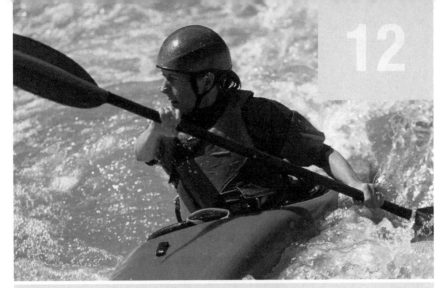

ulnar nerve entrapment

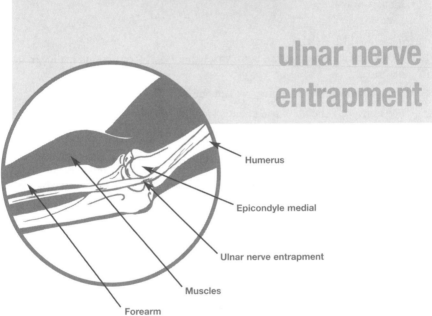

Humerus

Epicondyle medial

Ulnar nerve entrapment

Muscles

Forearm

6-POINT CONDITION STATEMENT

1. Definition

   A local traumatic condition to the inner (medial) elbow, causing acute or chronic nerve symptoms with pain and numbness.

2. Cause

   • Acute injury to the inner (medial) elbow at the "funny bone" (the ulnar nerve).

   • Chronic overuse in paddling activities of a malaligned elbow, causing stretching of the ulnar nerve.

3. Subjective Symptoms

- Pain at the elbow, radiating to the fourth and fifth fingers (ulnar nerve distribution).
- Numbness in the forearm, radiating to the fourth and fifth fingers.
- Weakness of fingers in severe cases.

4. Objective Findings

- Tenderness well localized to the inner elbow, directly on the ulnar nerve in the groove.
- Numbness and weakness of the hand.
- Motion intact.

5. Testing Procedures

- X-rays usually are negative, but a small spur may be present on the inner elbow.
- Bone scan and MRI generally are not helpful.
- EMG test may show chronic changes in the ulnar nerve.

6. Prognosis

Slow healing is generally possible with rest and by avoiding strenuous activities. Some chronic cases may need transfer and decompression of the nerve by surgical techniques.

10-POINT TREATMENT PLAN

1. Activity Levels

- Minimize overhead throwing and any activity that can torque the elbow.

2. Alternative Exercises

- Aerobic sports such as running, biking, and swimming are permitted.

3. Rehab Exercises

- See rehabilitation exercise program in Part IV of this book.
- Maintain range of motion and develop flexibility with strength using sandbags and tubing.

- Avoid excessive stretching or any symptoms that cause nerve symptoms.

4. Support

- Avoid any compressive, tight bandages around the elbow.
- Use foam pads to protect the elbow.

5. Thermal Treatment

- Local ice massage to reduce nerve inflammation.
- Heat to be used before activities for muscle relaxation.

6. Medication

- For oral medication, see "The 10-Point Treatment Plan" in Part II of this book.
- Anti-inflammatory medicine is sometimes helpful for reducing nerve inflammation. Some physicians recommend multivitamins for nerve regeneration.
- Local steroid injection is sometimes helpful for reducing inflammation.

7. Equipment

- Use paddling equipment with a large grip.

8. Nutrition

- Avoid weight gain during periods of inactivity.
- See nutrition suggestions in Part V of this book.

9. Fluids

- Maintain excellent hydration.

10. Surfaces

- Avoid running on hard surfaces to minimize jarring.
- Be careful of any twisting activities or falls.

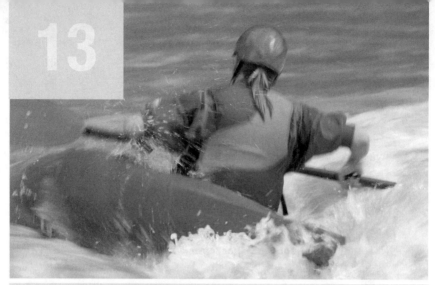

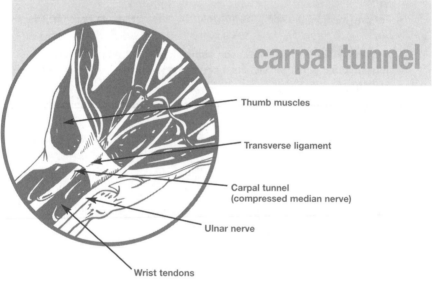

carpal tunnel

Thumb muscles

Transverse ligament

Carpal tunnel
(compressed median nerve)

Ulnar nerve

Wrist tendons

6-POINT CONDITION STATEMENT

1. Definition

A local inflammation characterized by pressure on or about the median nerve at the wrist, resulting in pain and numbness, especially when the wrist is in a flexed position.

2. Cause

- An acute injury, such as local trauma or compression, to the front (anterior) aspect of the wrist, causing local pain and swelling.

- A chronic, repetitive bent-wrist activity, such as in mountain climbing and paddling.

3. Subjective Symptoms

- Pain exists, especially in the radiation of the median nerve along the first three fingers and thumb, and especially at night.
- Strength may become reduced, especially in pinching.
- The wrist feels less pain when it is in an extended neutral position rather than a flexed position.

4. Objective Findings

- Local tenderness exists directly on the front of the wrist on the median nerve. When the nerve is trapped, radiating numbness develops in the thumb and index finger (a positive Tinel's sign).
- Sensory loss and motor weakness appear in the thumb and index finger.
- Symptoms are aggravated by placing the wrist in a flexed position.

5. Testing Procedures

- Routine x-rays generally are normal. Special views may show a small spur in the wrist.
- Bone scan may show inflammation if arthritis is present.
- EMG and nerve conduction studies are very helpful in detecting nerve damage.
- MRI may show compression of the nerve.

6. Prognosis

Healing potential is good, if the offending trauma can be reduced and local inflammation can be controlled. If pain and neurologic findings persist, surgical release of the ligament on the front of the wrist may be necessary.

10-POINT TREATMENT PLAN

1. Activity Levels

- Limit any wrist flexion activities, such as typing and repetitive movement.

2. Alternative Exercises

- Routine outdoor recreational activities, such as running, biking, and swimming, generally are not a problem.

- Excessive biking with the handlebar pressing on the wrist could cause a carpal tunnel.

3. Rehab Exercises

- See rehabilitation exercise program in Part IV of this book.

4. Support

- Use a wrist cockup splint to keep the wrist in a neutral position, especially at sleeping time.

5. Thermal Treatment

- Use local ice massage to reduce pain and swelling about the wrist.

6. Medication

- For oral medication, see "The 10-Point Treatment Plan" in Part II of this book.
- Simple anti-inflammatory medicine, such as aspirin or ibuprofen
- Local steroid injection to reduce inflammation and swelling.

7. Equipment

- Use proper work and sports splints to avoid excessive flexion of the wrist.
- Sleep with simple wrist splint.

8. Nutrition

- Avoid weight gain during periods of inactivity.
- See nutrition suggestions in Part V of this book.

9. Fluids

- Maintain excellent hydration.

10. Surfaces

- This usually is not a problem in carpal tunnel syndrome, but avoid running on concrete to reduce jarring to the body.

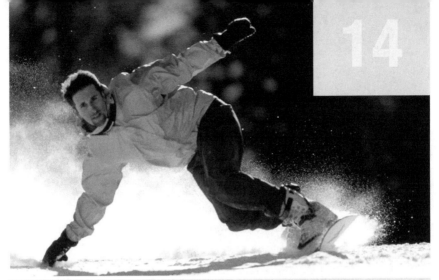

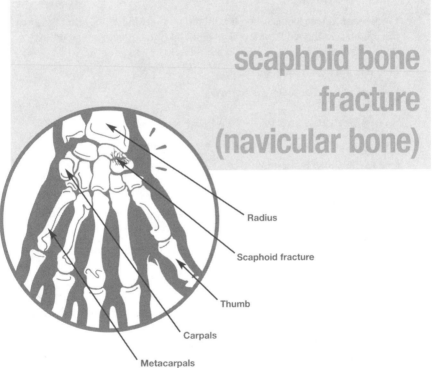

scaphoid bone fracture (navicular bone)

Radius

Scaphoid fracture

Thumb

Carpals

Metacarpals

6-POINT CONDITION STATEMENT

1. Definition

A traumatic condition of the thumb (radial) side from a fall on the hand, resulting in a fracture of the bone.

2. Cause

- An acute trauma to the wrist, generally from a fall (rarely a traumatic over-use condition).

3. Subjective Symptoms

- Immediate and intense pain following a fall; can be misinterpreted as a sprain.
- Swelling on the radial side of the wrist.
- Stiffness is very pronounced.

4. Objective Findings

- Tenderness is well localized on the thumb (radial) side of the wrist between the thumb and the wrist (anatomical snuff box, the space between the thumb tendons).
- Stiffness and loss of motion exist.
- Nerve and vascular testing is normal.

5. Testing Procedures

- X-rays should be examined carefully for a fracture of the scaphoid.
- Initial x-rays may be normal.
- Bone scan in a few days will show a possible fracture of the bone.
- MRI may be helpful.
- If all tests are negative, but there is a strong clinical suspicion, you should be treated for a fractured scaphoid.

6. Prognosis

The most important part of the case is early diagnosis and immobilization. Immobilization in either a short- or long-arm cast is recommended. The blood flow to this bone is very poor at times, and eventually surgery with a bone graft may be indicated in a small percentage of cases. If not treated properly, degenerative arthritis of the wrist may form.

10-POINT TREATMENT PLAN

1. Activity Levels

- Complete rest with splinting and casting of the wrist is required.
- Walking and moderate running are permitted.

2. Alternative Exercises

- During the cast immobilization period, walking, swimming, and biking are allowed. During swimming, put a plastic bag over the cast.

3. Rehab Exercises

- See rehabilitation exercise program in Part IV of this book.
- During cast immobilization, maintain isometric muscle tightening, exercises, and mobilization of the shoulder.

4. Support

- During the first-aid period, splinting is indicated, followed by a cast. Some surgeons recommend a short-arm cast, while some prefer a long-arm cast.

5. Thermal Treatment

- Use local ice initially for pain and swelling.
- Heat is not indicated because of the fracture and because it may cause more swelling.

6. Medication

- For oral medication, see "The 10-Point Treatment Plan" in Part II of this book.
- During cast immobilization, aspirin or anti-inflammatory medication may be indicated to reduce pain and swelling.
- Steroid injection is not indicated.

7. Equipment

- During the cast phase, biking may be used to maintain aerobic exercise.

8. Nutrition

- Avoid weight gain during periods of inactivity.
- See nutrition suggestions in Part V of this book.

9. Fluids

- Maintain excellent hydration.

10. Surfaces

- Hiking or running on nonjarring surfaces is indicated during the cast immobilization period.

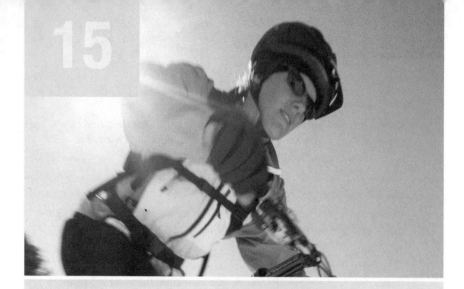

ulnar neuritis (biker's wrist)

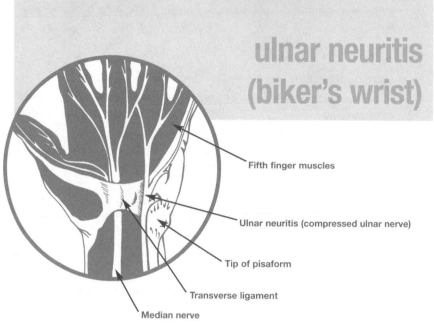

Fifth finger muscles

Ulnar neuritis (compressed ulnar nerve)

Tip of pisaform

Transverse ligament

Median nerve

6-POINT CONDITION STATEMENT

1. Definition

A local traumatic condition, usually seen in bicyclists, due to local pressure on the ulnar aspect (little finger side) of the wrist, resulting in pain and numbness in the fourth and fifth fingers.

2. Cause

- Acute violent trauma to the wrist in a fall or a direct hit on the ulnar aspect of the wrist.

- Chronic pressure in biking from leaning forward on the handlebar, with direct pressure on the ulnar aspect of the wrist.

3. Subjective Symptoms

- Pain in the wrist radiating to the fourth and fifth fingers.
- Numbness in the fourth and fifth fingers (ulnar nerve distribution) during biking.
- Weakness of the finger musculature.

4. Objective Findings

- Tenderness localized at the ulnar aspect of the wrist.
- Radiating numbness when the nerve is pressed or trapped (positive Tinel's sign).
- Sensory loss in the fourth and fifth fingers.
- Weakness of the small muscles of the hand, especially in the fourth and fifth fingers.

5. Testing Procedures

- X-rays usually are normal, but a small spur may be present.
- Bone scan is normal.
- MRI may show compression of the nerve.

6. Prognosis

Healing and reduction of pain occur with change in pressure, padding of the wrist, and conservative measures. Some cases may require a local injection of steroid along the nerve. Surgery is possible but rarely done.

10-POINT TREATMENT PLAN

1. Activity Levels

- Reduce the amount of biking and pressure on the wrist.

2. Alternative Exercises

- Hiking, running, and swimming are permissible.

3. Rehab Exercises

- See rehabilitation exercise program in Part IV of this book.
- Maintain muscle strength and hand grips.

4. Support

- Padding of the bicycle handle and biking gloves.

5. Thermal Treatment

- Local ice after biking to reduce pain and numbness.

6. Medication

- For oral medication, see "The 10-Point Treatment Plan" in Part II of this book.
- If pain persists, local injection of steroid.

7. Equipment

- Biking gloves that have special protection on the ulnar aspect of the wrist.
- Padded handlebars.
- Bicycle with an upright position, such as a mountain bike.

8. Nutrition

- Avoid weight gain during periods of inactivity.
- See nutrition suggestions in Part V of this book.

9. Fluids

- Maintain excellent hydration.

10. Surfaces

- Bicycle on smooth surfaces, and avoid any bouncing and rough terrain.

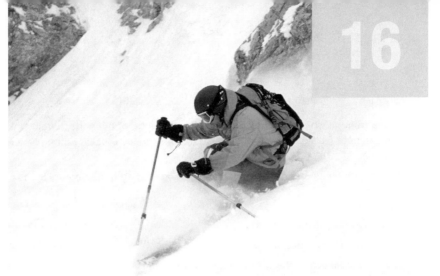

extensor tendon tear (baseball finger)

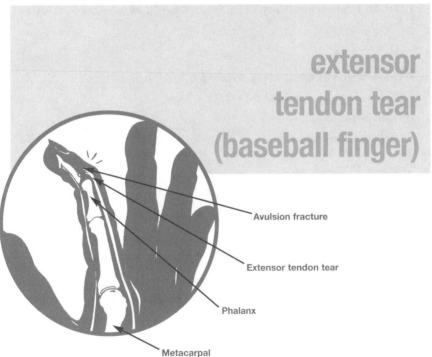

Avulsion fracture

Extensor tendon tear

Phalanx

Metacarpal

6-POINT CONDITION STATEMENT

1. Definition

A traumatic condition caused by direct, violent flexion to the tip of the finger, resulting in a tear of the tendon due to falling on an outstretched hand, such as in skiing, causing an acute flexion of the distal finger.

2. Cause

- Acute trauma, which hits and suddenly flexes the tip of the finger, tearing the extensor (straightening) tendon and in some cases breaking off a piece of bone.
- Chronic repetitive bending in an elderly person leading to microtears in the tendon.

3. Subjective Symptoms

- Sudden pain at the tip of the finger (dorsal aspect).
- Swelling localized to the extensor side of the finger.
- Inability to straighten the tip of the finger; fingertip appears bent (mallet finger).

4. Objective Findings

- Tenderness is localized to the dorsal tip of the finger.
- Local swelling is present at the tip of the finger.
- Weakness in extension.
- Nerve exam is normal.

5. Testing Procedures

- X-rays are normal if the tendon alone is torn. A bone injury may appear if a fracture is present.
- Bone scan and MRI are not needed.

6. Prognosis

Early treatment and diagnosis are vital to restoring tendon function. Splinting, casting, or pinning with open surgery may be chosen, depending on the extent of injury and the philosophy of the surgeon.

10-POINT TREATMENT PLAN

1. Activity Levels

- The hand must be rested to avoid further displacement of the fracture.

2. Alternative Exercises

- Running and biking are permitted to maintain aerobic fitness.

3. Rehab Exercises

- See rehabilitation exercise program in Part IV of this book.
- During periods of splinting, maintain upper-body strength and flexibility.

4. Support

- Keep the finger splinted in extension either with a tongue blade or a plastic, commercially prepared extension splint. This is required for 4 to 8 weeks.

5. Thermal Treatment

- Local ice to reduce pain and swelling.

6. Medication

- For oral medication, see "The 10-Point Treatment Plan" in Part II of this book.

7. Equipment

- The finger should be splinted promptly in extension (straight).

8. Nutrition

- Avoid weight gain during periods of inactivity.
- See nutrition suggestions in Part V of this book.

9. Fluids

- Maintain excellent hydration.

10. Surfaces

- Activities should be done on a nonskid surface to prevent falling on an outstretched hand.

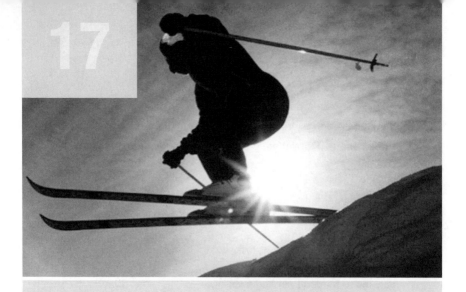

ruptured ulnar collateral ligament (skier's thumb)

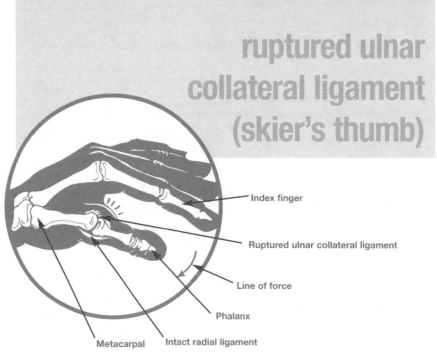

Index finger

Ruptured ulnar collateral ligament

Line of force

Phalanx

Metacarpal   Intact radial ligament

6-POINT CONDITION STATEMENT

1. Definition

A traumatic condition caused when a skier's outstretched hand falls onto a ski pole, resulting in a tear of the thumb ligament. Produces an unstable thumb and can lead to permanent disability.

2. Cause

- An acute tear of the ulnar ligament at the base of the thumb, usually in skiing, with the thumb bent outward from falling on the handle of the ski pole.
- Chronic stretching of the ligament from repeated minor stresses to the thumb.

3. Subjective Symptoms

- Sudden pain at the base of the thumb during a fall.
- Inability to sustain a pinch between the thumb and the index finger.
- Local swelling at the base of the thumb.
- Nerve symptoms are rare.

4. Objective Findings

- Instability at the base of the thumb with manual testing.
- Tenderness is localized at the ulnar aspect (small finger side) of the thumb.
- Swelling is localized at the ulnar aspect of the thumb.
- Nerve exam is normal.

5. Testing Procedures

- X-rays are normal; may be associated with a small fracture along the ligament.
- Stress x-rays are very helpful for showing instability (the physician manually attempts to displace the joint).
- Bone scan is not needed.
- MRI is not needed but could show the ligament tear.

6. Prognosis

Prompt treatment is very important. If misdiagnosed as a simple sprain and not treated properly, the injury could result in permanent instability and disability, leaving the hand with a weak pinch and pain. Early splinting, casting, and possibly surgery are recommended.

10-POINT TREATMENT PLAN

1. Activity Levels

- Stop skiing at first sign of injury, and seek proper treatment and diagnosis.

- During casting, light aerobic activities, such as light skiing, can be maintained if a proper protective splint has been applied.

2. Alternative Exercises

- Other activities such as biking, swimming, and running can be done.
- Upper-body weight lifting for flexibility and strength can be done.

3. Rehab Exercises

- See rehabilitation exercise program in Part IV of this book.
- During splinting and casting, maintain grip strength with isometric exercises for the hand.

4. Support

- Initially, the thumb should be properly splinted and casted until the extent of the instability and disability can be assessed.
- Use a protective thumb splint when returning to outdoor recreational activities.

5. Thermal Treatment

- Use local ice to reduce pain and swelling.
- Heat, which may cause more swelling and make casting difficulty, should not be used because of the severity of the injury.

6. Medication

- For oral medication, see "The 10-Point Treatment Plan" in Part II of this book.

7. Equipment

- Avoid ski pole straps that wrap around the thumb.
- Use ski poles that have plastic grips that fit around the wrist and hand.

8. Nutrition

- Avoid weight gain during periods of inactivity.
- See nutrition suggestions in Part V of this book.

9. Fluids

- Maintain excellent hydration.

10. Surfaces

- When returning to skiing, avoid hard moguls and hard bouncing until adequate strength has been regained.

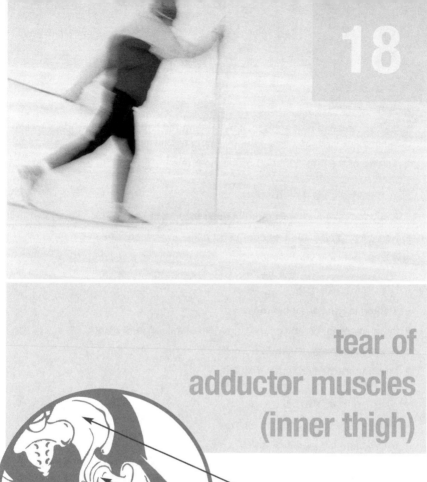

tear of adductor muscles (inner thigh)

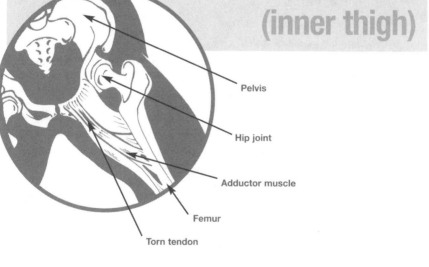

Pelvis

Hip joint

Adductor muscle

Femur

Torn tendon

6-POINT CONDITION STATEMENT

1. Definition

A traumatic muscle condition characterized by tearing or rupture of the adductor longus muscle (an inner muscle of the thigh that attaches to the pubic bone), resulting in local pain and limp.

2. Cause

- Sudden twisting and abduction (spreading the legs) in a high-impact twisting activity, such as cross-country skiing or downhill skiing.
- Tearing of the muscle group of the inner thigh.

3. Subjective Symptoms

- A sudden pain and pulling of the inner muscle of the thigh.
- Nerve symptoms such as numbness generally are not present.
- A limp, possibly very pronounced, and progressive swelling.

4. Objective Findings

- Marked restriction of hip motion.
- Local swelling, bleeding, and hematoma (collection of blood).
- Neurologic exam usually is normal.
- Muscle defects are sometimes felt.

5. Testing Procedures

- Initial x-rays are usually normal.
- Nerve tests are usually normal.
- Specialized testing, such as MRI, generally is not indicated but may show a muscle defect.
- After several months, x-rays may show muscle calcification.

6. Prognosis

If tearing is in the muscle belly, healing may occur within weeks. If tearing is in the tendon where it attaches to the bone, healing may take months. Surgery rarely is necessary to repair the defect. Slow but progressive rehabilitation can be expected. Return to outdoor recreational activities may take several months, depending on the extent of the tear.

10-POINT TREATMENT PLAN

1. Activity Levels

- Straight activities are best, as dictated by the pain.
- Avoid twisting and sudden cutting maneuvers during the first several weeks of rehabilitation.

2. Alternative Exercises

- Walking, swimming, and biking are satisfactory when the pain is less intense.
- Run in a swimming pool for early rehabilitation.

3. Rehab Exercises

- See rehabilitation exercise program in Part IV of this book.
- Rest is the best initial treatment.
- If pain is mild, early walking, swimming, and biking are satisfactory.
- Isometric exercises with simple weights are helpful for maintaining muscle mass.
- As pain gradually subsides, more aggressive muscle rehabilitation using an isokinetic exercise machine may be helpful.

4. Support

- Wrapping the thigh, taping the thigh, or using a special elastic wrap on the upper thigh is helpful.
- Be careful with compression if bleeding and swelling are pronounced.

5. Thermal Treatment

- Because of the initial pain and swelling, local ice massage is the best treatment.
- Local heat after several days reduces muscle spasms.

6. Medication

- For oral medication, see "The 10-Point Treatment Plan" in Part II of this book.
- After several weeks and if a local trigger point is present, an injection of Xylocaine and steroid may be of help.

7. Equipment

- Good supportive shoes are necessary for early walking.
- Thigh wraps are helpful for maintaining muscle support and minimizing swelling.

8. Nutrition

- Avoid weight gain during periods of inactivity.
- See nutrition suggestions in Part V of this book.

9. Fluids

- Maintain excellent hydration.

10. Surfaces

- Avoid impact and twisting activities early.
- Avoid hills and rough terrain.
- Stay on blacktop and bicycle paths for exercise.

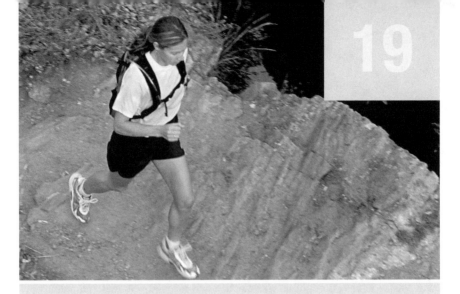

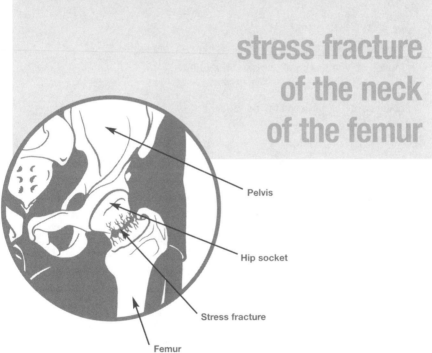

stress fracture
of the neck
of the femur

Pelvis

Hip socket

Stress fracture

Femur

6-POINT CONDITION STATEMENT

1. Definition

An overuse condition characterized by a localized weakening and cracking of the hipbone, due to repetitive lower extremity activities such as prolonged running on hard surfaces. Potentially a very serious problem that may require surgery if displacement of fracture is suspected or imminent.

2. Cause

- A prolonged running program on hard surfaces in a thin person, often a young woman, who is overtraining and losing weight.

3. Subjective Symptoms

- Progressive pain on the side, posterior aspect of the hip, or groin, with radiation into the inner thigh.
- Numbness and tingling usually are not present.
- Muscle spasm is present in some cases and often confused with simple muscle strain.
- Pain is usually brought on by activities and relieved with rest and sitting.

4. Objective Findings

- Limp is present, especially with hopping and running.
- Motion is guarded on hip flexion and rotation.
- Neurologic exam is normal.
- Local bone tenderness may be present.

5. Testing Procedures

- Initial x-rays may be normal, but a high index of suspicion should be present.
- Repeat x-rays should be done if pain persists. All persistent pain in the hip should be x-rayed to rule out a hip stress fracture because of the serious risk of displacement of fracture.
- Bone scan is very helpful in the early phases.
- MRI test may be positive and may show the fracture.
- EMG and nerve testing are normal.

6. Prognosis

Generally good, if rest is prescribed to allow the bone to heal. It may take 3 months for the fracture to heal. During this period, walking, swimming, and biking are permissible. Some surgeons recommend pinning of the fracture in a highly active individual.

10-POINT TREATMENT PLAN

1. Activity Levels

- Avoid any impact or twisting activity. Err on the side of overresting.
- As pain subsides, gradually increase walking, swimming, and biking.

2. Alternative Exercises

- Running in a swimming pool is allowed.
- Upper-body strengthening is allowed.
- Progress from walking, through race walking, to jogging.

3. Rehab Exercises

- See rehabilitation exercise program in Part IV of this book.
- Rest is especially indicated.
- Avoid any activities that cause pain.
- If walking, swimming, and biking are painless, they may be done with moderation.
- Maintain muscle strengthening with simple free weights.

4. Support

- The main help is emotional support from family, friends, and coaches.
- Athletes with this injury become frustrated and depressed rapidly.
- Braces about the hip are not helpful.

5. Thermal Treatment

- Ice and heat generally are not helpful. Rest is the key.
- If muscle spasm is present, heat can be tried.

6. Medication

- For oral medication, see "The 10-Point Treatment Plan" in Part II of this book.

7. Equipment

- Avoid any shoes that break down easily.
- Use stable shoes with excellent shock-absorbing qualities.
- Nonimpact exercise machines are permitted if there is no pain.

8. Nutrition

- Avoid weight gain during periods of inactivity.
- See nutrition suggestions in Part V of this book.
- Women who are not menstruating properly should consult a gynecologist who is knowledgeable in sports for possible estrogen therapy.

9. Fluids

- Maintain excellent hydration.

10. Surfaces

- Avoid any hills or firm surfaces during rehabilitation.
- Stay on blacktop and bicycle paths.
- Avoid any surfaces that cause pain.

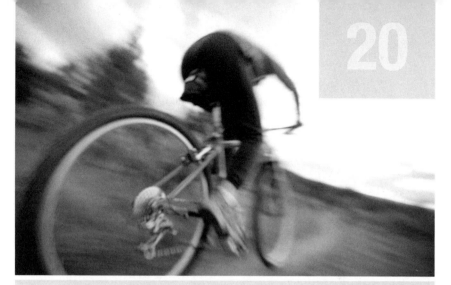

trochanteric bursitis

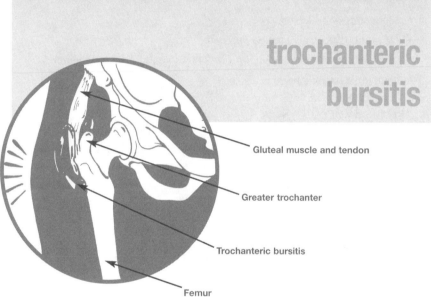

Gluteal muscle and tendon

Greater trochanter

Trochanteric bursitis

Femur

6-POINT CONDITION STATEMENT

1. Definition

Localized inflammation on the outer (lateral) side of the hip, characterized by local pain and limp, and common in aerobic activities.

2. Cause

- Long-distance running and biking, as well as cross-country skiing, cause the muscle tendons to rub over the side of the hip bone, leading to irritation of the bursa.

- May have leg alignment problems (knock-knee), and shoes may have worn excessively on the lateral heel.

3. Subjective Symptoms

- Localized pain exists on the side of the hip.
- Local swelling may be present.
- Numbness and tingling are not present.
- Pain is relieved with rest.
- Sneezing and coughing are not painful.

4. Objective Findings

- Slight limp with running.
- Hip motions possibly may be guarded.
- Local tenderness directly on the side of the hip (trochanteric region).
- Neurologic exam is normal.

5. Testing Procedures

- X-rays usually are normal but may show soft-tissue calcifications.
- Specialized tests such as MRI, CAT scan, myelogram, and EMG are not necessary.
- Bone scan may be positive.

6. Prognosis

Healing generally occurs after initial rest. Symptoms may linger for several months. Surgery rarely is necessary: Sometimes the bursa has to be excised and the tendon divided surgically, but this is unusual.

10-POINT TREATMENT PLAN

1. Activity Levels

- Avoid extreme twisting during running.
- Maintain progressive straight aerobic activities, such as moderate running and biking.

2. Alternative Exercises

- Race walking, biking, and running in a swimming pool.

3. Rehab Exercises

- See rehabilitation exercise program in Part IV of this book.
- Extreme rest is not necessary. Let pain be the guide.
- Moderate running, biking, and swimming are very helpful.
- Avoid extreme long-distance running during periods of pain.
- Do simple weight lifting to strengthen the front and side muscles.
- Progressive isokinetic exercises are helpful, but avoid torqueing the hip excessively.

4. Support

- Local wrap generally is not helpful.

5. Thermal Treatment

- Local ice massage is very helpful for reducing the swelling of the bursa.
- If muscle spasm is present, heat may be used.

6. Medication

- For oral medication, see "The 10-Point Treatment Plan" in Part II of this book.
- Steroid injection is sometimes helpful for reducing the swelling in the bursa.

7. Equipment

- Avoid any lateral heel wear on the shoe. Wear firm-heeled shoes.

8. Nutrition

- Avoid weight gain during periods of inactivity.
- See nutrition suggestions in Part V of this book.

9. Fluids

- Maintain excellent hydration.

10. Surfaces

- Avoid banks and hills and anything that will torque the hips.
- Stay on blacktop and bicycle paths for exercise.

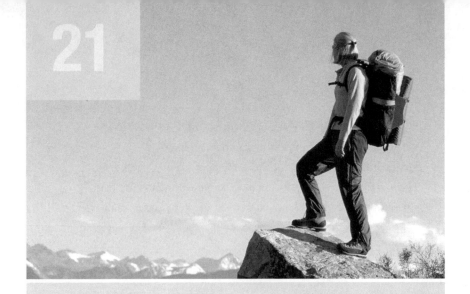

myositis ossificans, heterotopic bone formation

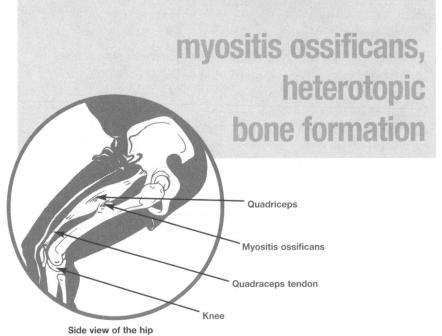

Quadriceps

Myositis ossificans

Quadraceps tendon

Knee

Side view of the hip

6-POINT CONDITION STATEMENT

1. Definition

A chronic soft-tissue inflammatory-traumatic condition with tearing and bleeding in the thigh muscle, resulting in abnormal scarring and extra bone formation (myositis ossificans) directly inside the muscle. Generally starts as a simple muscle tear or bleed caused by direct trauma or tear during mountain or rock climbing. If muscle is not immobilized and rested, bone will form in it.

2. Cause

- A sudden impact or tearing of the quadriceps muscle.
- Lack of immobilization and rest in an injured muscle.

3. Subjective Symptoms

- Persistent pain several months after an injury to the thigh muscle.
- Tightness and stiffness of the thigh muscle, with limitation of knee and hip motion.
- Stability is excellent.
- A firm mass is felt in some cases.

4. Objective Findings

- Well-localized tenderness and thickening of the muscle.
- Restriction in thigh and knee motion.
- A tender, swollen mass may be felt.

5. Testing Procedures

- X-rays show calcification and bone formation in the muscle.
- A bone scan and MRI may further document the problem.
- Arthroscopy is not helpful.

6. Prognosis

Aggressive physical therapy and many months of healing are required. Sometimes ultrasound therapy helps to speed healing and reduce the inflammation. Surgery is rarely indicated. The long-term function is good, but the healing period may be prolonged.

10-POINT TREATMENT PLAN

1. Activity Levels

- Let pain be the guide. Injury is caused by excessive activity during pain.

2. Alternative Exercises

- Running, biking, swimming, and running in a swimming pool are all excellent ways of maintaining muscle function and aerobic activity.

- Forceful, heavy weight lifting is not indicated until the pain gradually subsides.

3. Rehab Exercises

- See rehabilitation exercise program in Part IV of this book.
- Straight-leg raising and bent-knee isometric exercises are indicated once the pain starts to subside.
- Do not force exercises or stretching; this may cause more inflammation.

4. Support

- Wrapping the thigh may help to maintain muscle compression and support.
- Wear a protective rubber pad on the thigh to prevent impact.

5. Thermal Treatment

- Ice during the acute muscle tear and bleed.
- In the chronic state, local heat to reduce muscle inflammation, along with a program of gentle exercise and rest.

6. Medication

- For oral medication, see"The 10-Point Treatment Plan" in Part II of this book.
- Local steroid injection may be helpful in the late phase of recovery.

7. Equipment

- Good shock-absorbing shoes.
- Isokinetic machines for gentle strength and flexibility.

8. Nutrition

- Avoid weight gain during periods of inactivity.
- See nutrition suggestions in Part V of this book.

9. Fluids

- Maintain excellent hydration.

10. Surfaces

- Avoid running on hills or anything that excessively flexes the thigh.

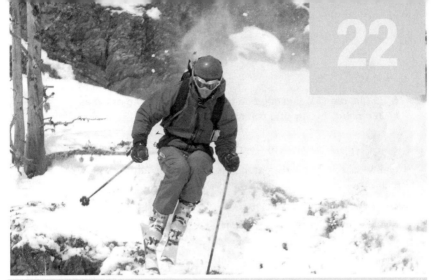

quadriceps muscle tear

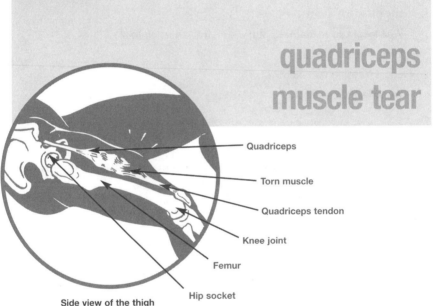

Quadriceps

Torn muscle

Quadriceps tendon

Knee joint

Femur

Hip socket

Side view of the thigh

6-POINT CONDITION STATEMENT

1. Definition

A traumatic muscle condition characterized by a sudden tearing of the muscle on the front of the thigh between the kneecap and hip joint, resulting in severe pain, limp, and inability to extend the knee.

2. Cause

- An acute contraction or sudden flexion of the thigh muscle, overloading the muscle strength and causing a tear of the quadriceps muscle, often just above the kneecap.

- A chronic repetitive tearing due to excessive jumping or excessive overload, as in running, biking, and surfing.

3. Subjective Symptoms

- Well-localized tenderness at the muscle–tendon junction, generally 2 to 3 inches above the kneecap.
- Local swelling in some cases.
- A sensation of giving way due to muscle weakness, especially if there is a complete tear of the muscle.
- Jumping and kicking are very painful.

4. Objective Findings

- Well-localized tenderness at the site of the muscle tear.
- Limp may be present.
- Local swelling and bleeding.
- Weakness on extension of the knee.

5. Testing Procedures

- Routine x-rays generally are normal.
- MRI usually is not necessary but may show a tear of the muscle or tendon.
- Arthroscopy is not helpful.

6. Prognosis

Incomplete tears usually heal. If the diagnosis is not made initially and activity persists, calcification (called heterotopic bone formation or myositis ossificans) may form in the tendon. If there is a complete tear of the muscle–tendon junction, open surgical repair may be indicated.

10-POINT TREATMENT PLAN

1. Activity Levels

- For a severe tear, surgery and rest are generally indicated.
- For incomplete tears, slow, gradual walking, biking, and running are permissible.
- Avoid jumping and kicking.

2. Alternative Exercises

- Early in recovery, swimming is permissible, especially if the leg is straight.
- Gradually progress to walking, biking, and light running.
- Hard jumping and kicking are the last activities.

3. Rehab Exercises

- See rehabilitation exercise program in Part IV of this book.
- Straight-leg-raising exercises and isometric contraction of the muscle are permissible early if no major tear exists.
- In a few weeks, as pain subsides, start gentle flexion exercises using isokinetic machines. Let pain be the guide.

4. Support

- For an incomplete tear, wrap the thigh using large elastic wraps.
- A protective rubber pad on the front of the thigh helps prevent impact injuries.

5. Thermal Treatment

- Local ice massage and compression.
- Heat in a few days as pain and swelling subsides.

6. Medication

- For oral medication, see "The 10-Point Treatment Plan" in Part II of this book.
- After several months, a local steroid injection may be helpful at trigger points.

7. Equipment

- Generally, sports equipment is not a factor.
- Keep bicycle seat high.

8. Nutrition

- Avoid weight gain during periods of inactivity.
- See nutrition suggestions in Part V of this book.

9. Fluids

- Maintain excellent hydration.

10. Surfaces

- Avoid running on hills and climbing stairs.
- Do activities on straight paths.

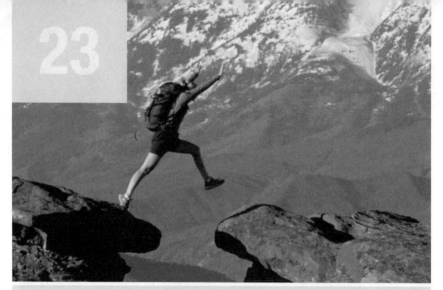

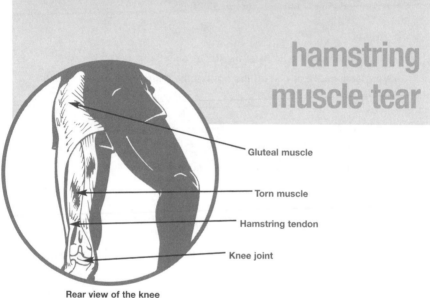

hamstring
muscle tear

Gluteal muscle

Torn muscle

Hamstring tendon

Knee joint

Rear view of the knee

6-POINT CONDITION STATEMENT

1. Definition

A traumatic muscle condition characterized by a sudden tearing of the muscles of the posterior or hamstring. The tear is usually located in the central portion of the thigh or the tendons at the knee or hip. Injury results in acute localized pain, limp, and inability to run.

2. Cause

- A sudden extension or violent jumping activity, overloading the muscle and causing an acute tear.

- A chronic, repetitive overuse condition due to tight muscle associated with running, biking, and jumping.

3. Subjective Symptoms

- Well-localized sharp pain in the muscle belly or pain near the knee or hip.
- Local swelling and bleeding are present in some cases.
- Stability is good, but there is pain with jumping.

4. Objective Findings

- Well-localized tenderness.
- Well-localized swelling and bruising.
- Pain on stretching the hamstring.
- Neurologic exam is normal.

5. Testing Procedures

- Routine x-rays are normal.
- Arthrogram is not helpful.
- MRI usually is not necessary but may show a tear of the tendon.

6. Prognosis

Healing is often more prolonged with the hamstring tendon than with the quadriceps muscle in the front. The pain may persist for many months because of tight hamstring muscles. Surgery rarely is indicated, except for complete severe tear of the hamstring tendon where it attaches to the knee.

10-POINT TREATMENT PLAN

1. Activity Levels

- Early biking, swimming, and walking are satisfactory.
- As pain gradually subsides, intense running or biking is permissible.
- Jumping and rapid twisting are the last activities to be considered.

2. Alternative Exercises

- Running in a swimming pool is an excellent way of maintaining aerobic activity and reducing strain on the hamstring tendon.

- Avoid violent kicking.

3. Rehab Exercises

- See rehabilitation exercise program in Part IV of this book.
- Rest is indicated at first.
- Do isometric exercises with the leg straight for early pain.
- As pain subsides, gradually return to flexion and stretching exercises with isokinetic machines.

4. Support

- Wrap the thigh with elastic wraps, which will help reduce the pull on the inflamed muscle and tendon.

5. Thermal Treatment

- Ice massage to reduce pain and swelling.
- Local heat after several days to reduce muscle soreness.

6. Medication

- For oral medication, see "The 10-Point Treatment Plan" in Part II of this book.
- If pain persists after several months, a local steroid injection may be of help in an inflamed area.

7. Equipment

- Keep the heel elevated with a very thick-heeled running shoe to reduce the hamstring pull.
- Use machine (biking, rowing) to maintain muscle flexibility and strength.

8. Nutrition

- Avoid weight gain during periods of inactivity.
- See nutrition suggestions in Part V of this book.

9. Fluids

- Maintain excellent hydration.

10. Surfaces

- Avoid hills and twisting and activities.
- Run on soft surfaces, such as blacktop or bicycle paths.

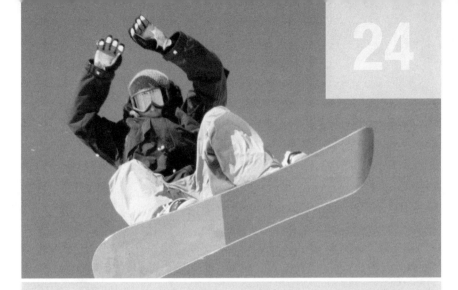

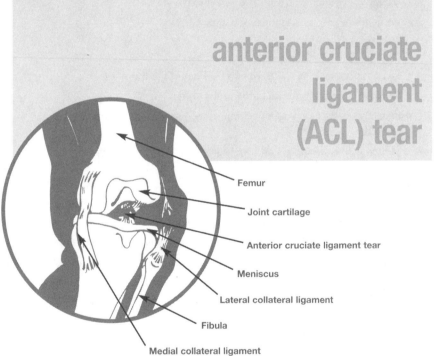

anterior cruciate
ligament
(ACL) tear

Femur

Joint cartilage

Anterior cruciate ligament tear

Meniscus

Lateral collateral ligament

Fibula

Medial collateral ligament

6-POINT CONDITION STATEMENT

1. Definition

A traumatic tearing of the main central ligament of the knee (anterior cruciate ligament, ACL), characterized by sudden twisting, giving way, and falling to the ground, causing a shifting and a "pop," with resulting disability. Can be serious condition requiring proper diagnosis, not just treated as knee pain.

2. Cause

- Acute twist and falling injury in jumping and twisting activities, such as snowboarding and skiing.
- Chronic repeated microtrauma of many knee sprains, leading to progressive tearing from incomplete to complete disruption.

3. Subjective Symptoms

- Pain on the front or back of the knee.
- Swelling within 1 to 3 hours as blood accumulates.
- A sensation of giving way and a shifting of the knee.
- Motion is restricted as pain and swelling develop.
- Progressive limp and inability to jump.

4. Objective Findings

- Local tenderness on the front inner aspect of the knee.
- Swelling is present due to blood in the knee.
- Instability tests (such as a Lachman's test) show drawer and pivot shift positive.
- Motion is very restricted and limited in flexion and extension.

5. Testing Procedures

- Initial x-rays are normal but may show a small associated fracture. Chronic cases may show early signs of degenerative arthritis.
- MRI shows characteristic changes in the ligament and the meniscus.
- Arthrogram does not help to show to show the tear of the ligament but may show associated tears of the menisci.
- Arthroscopy is very diagnostic but should be reserved for severe cases.

6. Prognosis

Tears of the anterior cruciate ligament are an enigma. Healing of the torn ligament is unpredictable because of poor blood supply to the ligament. The prognosis depends on the extent of instability and the activity level of the individual. There are many philosophies of treatment, ranging from muscle rehabilitation to sophisticated braces to complex surgical procedures. Individuals should expect many months of rehabilitation before returning to twisting activities.

10-POINT TREATMENT PLAN

1. Activity Levels

- After the injury, rest is mandatory, but upper-body aerobic exercises are permissible.

2. Alternative Exercises

- During rehabilitation, twisting activities should be avoided.
- Exercises that develop the thigh muscle should be done. You may progress from walking, biking, and running in a swimming pool to jogging over a 3- to 6-month period.

3. Rehab Exercises

- See rehabilitation exercise program in Part IV of this book.
- For the acute tear, isometric exercises can be done to maintain muscle strength.
- During the rehabilitation phase, particular emphasis on the hamstring muscle is very important.

4. Support

- Depending on the extent of instability, simple to very complex custom-made braces are advisable for stabilizing the knee.
- Braces are very effective in supporting the knee but are not a substitute for muscle rehabilitation and modification of activity.

5. Thermal Treatment

- Use ice for the first few days to reduce pain and swelling.
- Heat should not be used because it may aggravate the swelling of the knee.
- During rehabilitation, heat helps to maintain muscle relaxation.

6. Medication

- For oral medication, see "The 10-Point Treatment Plan" inPart II of this book.

7. Equipment

- A good stabilizing shoe is very important for maintaining foot control during rehabilitation.

- Most exercise machines are satisfactory as long as they do not twist and torque the knee.

8. Nutrition

- Avoid weight gain during periods of inactivity.

- See nutrition suggestions in Part V of this book.

9. Fluids

- Maintain excellent hydration.

10. Surfaces

- Because of instability, curved rough surfaces should be avoided.

- Rough terrain must be avoided because it may cause more instability.

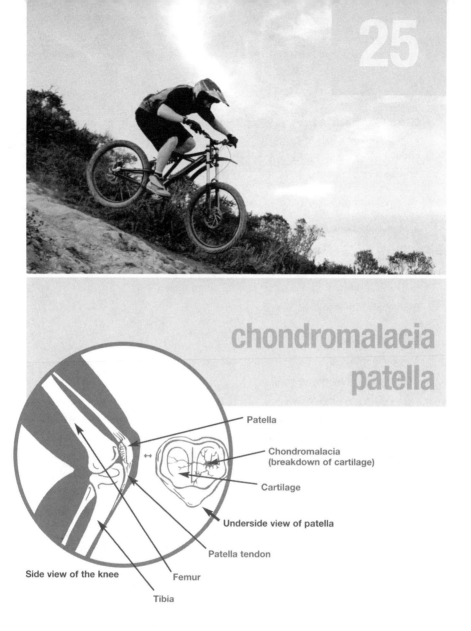

chondromalacia patella

Patella

Chondromalacia
(breakdown of cartilage)

Cartilage

Underside view of patella

Patella tendon

Side view of the knee

Femur

Tibia

6-POINT CONDITION STATEMENT

1. Definition

A traumatic or degenerative cartilage condition characterized by a local break-down of the undersurface of the cartilage, usually at the patella; can be an early localized form of osteoarthritis or degenerative arthritis.

2. Cause

- Direct local trauma, such as when the knee hits the dashboard in an automobile accident.
- Repeated bending microtrauma, especially if the joint is not aligned properly, as in trail running and mountain biking.

3. Subjective Symptoms

- Dull, aching pain, leading to sharp localized pain in the front of the knee
- Grinding sensation is frequently present.
- Swelling and fluid generally are not present.
- Stiffness in squatting, bending, and climbing stairs.
- Sensation of giving way.

4. Objective Findings

- Motion is intact.
- Stability of ligaments is good.
- Swelling is not present.
- Tenderness is localized to the patella joint.
- Patella maltracking is present (kneecap is not in proper alignment).
- Crepitation (grinding sensation) is felt.

5. Testing Procedures

- Gait analysis shows knock-knees or bowed legs with pronation (flat arches) of the feet.
- X-rays show slight spurring of the patellar joint and malalignment of the patella.
- Bone scan helps to show localized uptake and inflammation.
- MRI test is not very helpful.
- Arthroscopy is diagnostic but should be done only after failure of conservative treatment.

6. Prognosis

Good, but healing can be prolonged. Some cases progress and may need surgery in the form of arthroscopy or major open patella realignment.

10-POINT TREATMENT PLAN

1. Activity Levels

- Avoid bent-knee twisting activities, such as hard running up hills.
- Straight activities, such as biking with high seat, walking, and slow running, are best.

2. Alternative Exercises

- Swimming and running in a swimming pool are excellent aerobic alternatives.
- Avoid the breaststroke (the frog kick).

3. Rehab Exercises

- See rehabilitation exercise program in Part IV of this book.
- Straight-leg-raising exercises with 5- to 10-pound weights are allowed.

4. Support

- Use patella brace (an elastic sleeve with cutout for the patella).

5. Thermal Treatment

- Local ice massage is best.
- Heat for muscle spasm.

6. Medication

- For oral medication, see "The 10-Point Treatment Plan" in Part II of this book.
- Local steroid injections generally are not helpful.

7. Equipment

- Wear firm-heeled antipronation shoes.
- Consider custom-made orthotics (arch supports) for shoes.

8. Nutrition

- Avoid weight gain during periods of inactivity.
- See nutrition suggestions in Part V of this book.

9. Fluids

- Maintain excellent hydration.

10. Surfaces

- Avoid hills and banked tracks.
- Use flat, soft surfaces like blacktop or bicycle paths for exercises.

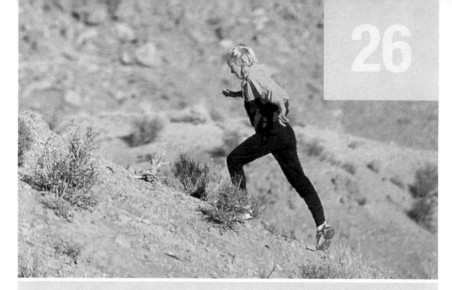

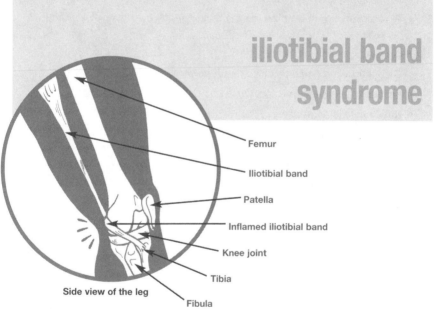

iliotibial band syndrome

Femur

Iliotibial band

Patella

Inflamed iliotibial band

Knee joint

Tibia

Side view of the leg

Fibula

6-POINT CONDITION STATEMENT

1. Definition

An overuse inflammatory condition of the outer (lateral) aspect of the knee, characterized by an ache and burning sensation during or after running, due to local friction of a tendon band as it rubs the outer bone of the knee (lateral condyle).

2. Cause

• Acute, local, direct trauma; a rare cause.

- Chronic, overuse microtrauma, usually in training in activities such as trail running and mountain biking. Pain is usually not disabling.

3. Subjective Symptoms

- Pain is well localized to the side of the knee on the outer flare of the bone.
- The pain may radiate up the side of the thigh to the hip.
- Swelling usually is not present.
- Motion is normal, but tightness may be perceived.
- Snapping may be present.

4. Objective Findings

- Tenderness is well localized to the band directly over the outer lateral condyle.
- Swelling generally is not present.
- Crepitation and noise usually are not present.
- Instability is not present.
- Knee exam is normal.
- Tightness of the lateral muscles may be present.

5. Testing Procedures

- X-rays generally are normal.
- Bone scan may be positive in chronic cases, showing bone inflammation.
- MRI is rarely indicated.
- Arthroscopy is not indicated.

6. Prognosis

Progressive healing occurs with simple reduction in activity and muscle rehabilitation. You may continue moderate biking and running during this condition. Surgery to split the tendon may be done in rare cases.

10-POINT TREATMENT PLAN

1. Activity Levels

- You do not have to stop running; simply reduce the intensity during periods of pain.

2. Alternative Exercises

- Biking and running in a swimming pool are excellent alternatives for the runner.
- Avoid running on hills.

3. Rehab Exercises

- See rehabilitation exercise program in Part IV of this book.
- Maintain muscle flexibility, endurance, speed, and strength, with particular emphasis on stretching the lateral muscles of the thigh and knee.

4. Support

- Simple elastic wrap or Neoprene wrap around the knee may be helpful.
- Avoid wraps that are too tight; they may lead to more friction.

5. Thermal Treatment

- Local ice massage directly after running.
- Heat massage to relax muscles before activities.

6. Medication

- For oral medication, see "The 10-Point Treatment Plan" in Part II of this book.
- In rare cases, a local steroid injection may be used after months of treatment to reduce local inflammation.

7. Equipment

- Work more on upper-body aerobic exercises, and rest the knee.
- Shoes tend to wear on the lateral side of the heel. Wear shoes that have firm outer heels to stabilize the heel during heel strike.

8. Nutrition

- Avoid weight gain during periods of inactivity.
- See nutrition suggestions in Part V of this book.

9. Fluids

- Maintain excellent hydration.

10. Surfaces

- Avoid running on hard, rough surfaces.

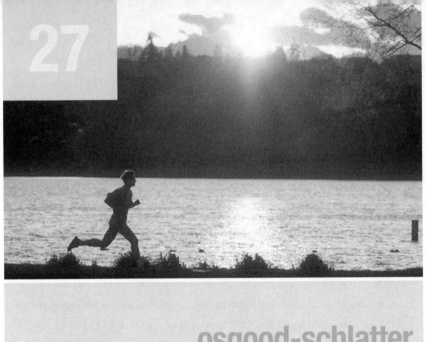

osgood-schlatter disease

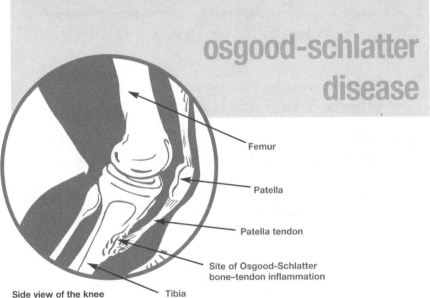

Femur

Patella

Patella tendon

Site of Osgood-Schlatter
bone–tendon inflammation

Side view of the knee   Tibia

6-POINT CONDITION STATEMENT

1. Definition

A traumatic tendon condition seen in adolescents ages 12 to 14. Condition characterized by pain where the tendon attaches to the shin bone (tibial tuberosity, a growth zone). Not really a disease.

2. Cause

- A sudden jump causing a local tearing of the growth zone where the tendon attaches.

- Chronic: repetitive jumping, running, and bending in a young, growing adolescent. Just as in "jumper's knee," may be aggravated by leg and foot imbalance or excessive running.

3. Subjective Symptoms

- Pain: a progressive ache below the knee in activities such as jumping and hard running.
- Swelling: a firm bump below the knee.
- Motion is intact.
- Nerve symptoms are not present.

4. Objective Findings

- Local tenderness at the tibial tuberosity.
- Bony, hard mass felt 1 to 2 inches below the kneecap.
- Knee exam is otherwise within normal limits.

5. Testing Procedures

- X-rays show a fragmentation and enlargement of the growth zone at the tibial tuberosity.
- Bone scan may show inflammation, but scan is rarely indicated.
- MRI is not indicated.
- Arthroscopy is not indicated.

6. Prognosis

Symptoms persist until growth stops at age 16 or 17. With decrease in activity, there is reduction in pain. There is no need to stop all activities. A bony bump may be permanent but not disabling. In rare cases, the bump needs to be removed surgically once growth ends. As an adult, the bump may be a problem in certain occupations, such as carpet laying and plumbing, that require kneeling.

10-POINT TREATMENT PLAN

1. Activity Levels

- Moderate reduction in activity is needed, but there is no need to stop activities. This is not a disease, nor is it a serious condition.

2. Alternative Exercises

- Try to avoid hard jumping activities.
- Moderate biking, swimming, and running are permitted.

3. Rehab Exercises

- See rehabilitation exercise program in Part IV of this book.
- Maintain flexibility, endurance, speed, and strength with moderate biking and weight lifting.

4. Support

- Simple elastic wrap or Neoprene sleeve around the knee will help reduce the pressure on the bone center.

5. Thermal Treatment

- Local ice massage after outdoor recreational activities.
- Heat before activities to relax muscles.

6. Medication

- For oral medication, see "The 10-Point Treatment Plan" in Part II of this book.
- Medications generally are not necessary, but acetaminophen (Tylenol) can be taken.

7. Equipment

- Use good stabilizing shoes to prevent foot imbalance.

8. Nutrition

- Avoid weight gain during periods of inactivity.
- See nutrition suggestions in Part V of this book.

9. Fluids

- Maintain excellent hydration.

10. Surfaces

- Trail running should be on soft surfaces without major hills.
- Avoid concrete for outdoor recreational activities.
- Avoid running on curved surfaces.

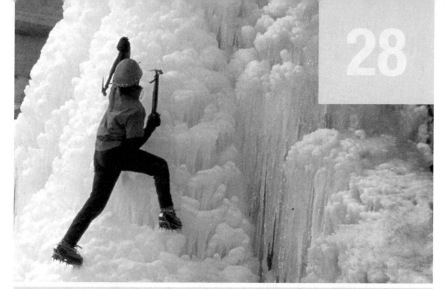

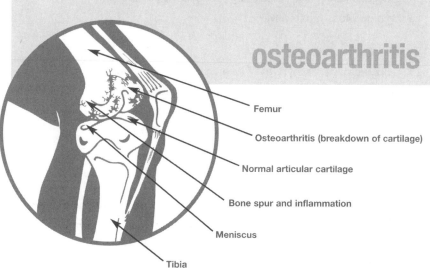

osteoarthritis

Femur

Osteoarthritis (breakdown of cartilage)

Normal articular cartilage

Bone spur and inflammation

Meniscus

Tibia

6-POINT CONDITION STATEMENT

1. Definition

A traumatic or degenerative condition of the cartilage of the knee joint, characterized by progressive wearing of the articular surface (hyaline cartilage). Progressive pain and stiffness result. Bone spur formation gives the condition the name osteoarthritis. Progressive deterioration because of poor circulation to cartilage.

2. Cause

- Acute: traumatic injury to the surface of the joint from an impact or a twisting injury.

- Chronic: years of microtrauma to a joint, especially if malalignment or instability is present, such as with a torn anterior cruciate ligament (ACL).
- Other causes: obesity, idiopathic (cause not known) changes, and hereditary factors.

3. Subjective Symptoms

- Pain and ache are present after activity. The pain may be delayed until the next day or night.
- Swelling may be present in or around the joint.
- A sensation of giving way may be present while climbing stairs.
- Crepitation and noise can be felt and heard by the patient.
- Limp develops progressively.

4. Objective Findings

- Tenderness is present directly on the joint and along bone spurs.
- Swelling and fluid accumulation can be perceived.
- Crepitation can be felt and heard by the patient.
- Stiffness and loss of motion are detected.
- Limp is present with weight bearing and jumping.

5. Testing Procedures

- Initial x-rays are normal, even though cartilage is wearing. As the condition worsens, x-rays reveal roughness, narrowing of joint line, and spur formation.
- Bone scan is very helpful for detecting bone inflammation.
- MRI shows tears of the meniscus and wearing of the cartilage.
- Arthroscopy will definitely show defects in the hyaline cartilage, but generally the test is not used early to establish the diagnosis. Arthroscopy may be helpful in treating moderate cases by smoothing roughened surfaces and removing loose bodies. The patient should be warned that in some cases arthroscopy may aggravate the problem with disappointing results.

6. Prognosis

Progressive deterioration of the joint will occur if you do not listen to your body. Pain indicates that progressive wearing is occurring. Reduce the intensity of activities until pain is minimal. Moderation of activity and intensity is very important. Twisting activities should be minimized. Nonimpact activities, such as biking, walking, and swimming, are satisfactory. Surgery, ranging from arthroscopy to eventual total joint replacement, may be required if the condition is very serious.

10-POINT TREATMENT PLAN

1. Activity Levels

- Nonimpact activities are best.
- Avoid any exercise that causes discomfort directly in the joint.

2. Alternative Exercises

- Swimming, biking, and walking are best in moderation.

3. Rehab Exercises

- See rehabilitation exercise program in Part IV of this book.
- Maintain muscle strength and flexibility with moderate, nonimpact exercises.
- Gentle weight lifting, swimming, and biking are permissible.

4. Support

- The best support is muscle development.
- During periods of pain and swelling, a simple elastic wrap or brace can be used around the inflamed joint.
- Use trekking/walking stick for limp to reduce stress on the joint. (See information on walking poles in Part V of this book.)

5. Thermal Treatment

- During period of acute pain and swelling, ice is preferred.
- Use heat for local muscle tightness and stiffness of the joint.

6. Medication

- For oral medication, see "The 10-Point Treatment Plan" in Part II of this book.
- Nonsteroidal anti-inflammatory medications may be prescribed by your physician.
- Local steroid injection and aspiration may be tried intermittently but should be kept to a minimum.

7. Equipment

- Use stable, firm-heeled shoes.
- Avoid equipment that excessively bends the joint.

8. Nutrition

- Avoid weight gain during periods of inactivity.
- See nutrition suggestions in Part V of this book.

9. Fluids

- Maintain excellent hydration.

10. Surfaces

- It is very important to avoid hard, rough surfaces during walking, running, and sports activities.

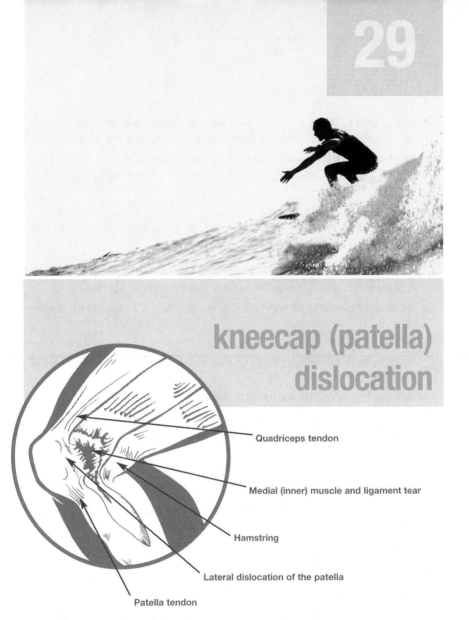

kneecap (patella) dislocation

Quadriceps tendon

Medial (inner) muscle and ligament tear

Hamstring

Lateral dislocation of the patella

Patella tendon

6-POINT CONDITION STATEMENT

1. Definition

A traumatic condition in which the kneecap (patella) slides or shifts to the outer (lateral) side of the knee, either momentarily (until the patella replaces itself) or for a prolonged period (until a physician reduces it).

2. Cause

- Acute: a fall or direct trauma to the front and inner side of the kneecap, resulting in tearing of the inner ligaments, which stabilize the patella.
- Chronic: usually in an adolescent female with malalignment (knock-knees) and lax ligaments, resulting in a shift of the patella in a twisting activity.

3. Subjective Symptoms

- Pain is localized to the front and inner side of the patella.
- Swelling of the knee is present due to bleeding.
- Kneecap is perceived to be out of place in some cases.
- A sensation of giving way is felt as the patella slides out of place.
- Grinding sensation is present because of injury to the surface of the patella.

4. Objective Findings

- Tenderness is localized to the inner side of the patella, where the ligaments are torn.
- Swelling from bleeding is present in the knee.
- A mass is perceived. Patella is out of place on the lateral side of the knee.
- Crepitation and noise are present from a possible fracture of the patella.

5. Testing Procedures

- X-ray may be normal if the patella has popped back in place.
- Malalignment of the patella with possible fracture may be noted on special patella views.
- Bone scan initially may be normal but later may be positive because of degenerative changes.
- MRI test is usually not helpful, but special techniques may show malalignment of the patella.
- Arthroscopy is usually not necessary to substantiate the diagnosis but may be helpful to show fractures of the patella surface.

6. Prognosis

In a male with acute trauma to the patella, spontaneous healing of the ligaments and muscles usually occurs without recurrence of the dislocation. In a female with laxity and malalignment, recurrent dislocation may occur, requiring limitation in outdoor recreational activities and possible surgery to realign the patella.

10-POINT TREATMENT PLAN

1. Activity Levels

- Rest the knee and avoid any flexion activities during the acute healing phase.

2. Alternative Exercises

- Upper-body exercises such as with an aerodyne bicycle are permitted. Biking with the good leg is permitted. Place the painful knee on a chair or on a bicycle bar.

3. Rehab Exercises

- See rehabilitation exercise program in Part IV of this book.
- Avoid any exercises that flex the knee and stress the patella.
- Maintain muscle quadriceps strength with straight-leg-raising exercises, and follow a patellar rehabilitation program.

4. Support

- The knee should be immobilized in extension (straight) for 2 to 4 weeks either in a cast or in a knee immobilizer.
- During the rehabilitation phase, special patella harnesses and braces help to maintain the proper position of the patella until muscle rehabilitation is complete.

5. Thermal Treatment

- Use ice daily to reduce pain and swelling.
- During the rehabilitation phase, heat may be used for muscle relaxation.

6. Medication

- For oral medication, see "The 10-Point Treatment Plan" in Part II of this book.
- The knee may need to be aspirated of the blood and possibly injected with an anti-inflammatory medication because of recurrent fluid formation.

7. Equipment

- During the initial healing phase, avoid any exercise that flexes the knees—for example, biking, running, or heavy weight lifting.

8. Nutrition

- Avoid weight gain during periods of inactivity.
- See nutrition suggestions in Part V of this book.

9. Fluids

- Maintain excellent hydration.

10. Surfaces

- During rehabilitation, do light sports on nonskid surfaces.
- Biking and running should be on smooth, soft surfaces that will not jar or twist the knee.

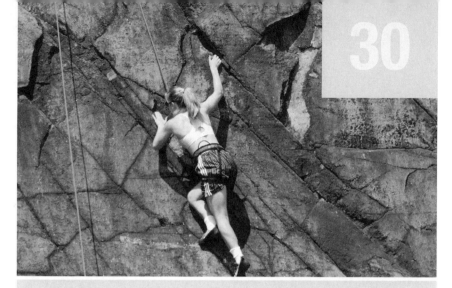

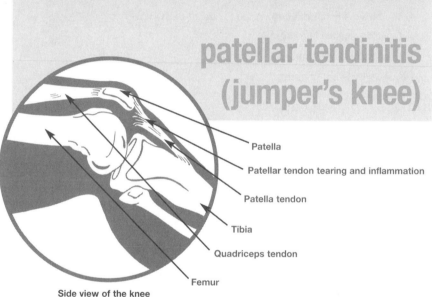

patellar tendinitis (jumper's knee)

Patella

Patellar tendon tearing and inflammation

Patella tendon

Tibia

Quadriceps tendon

Femur

Side view of the knee

6-POINT CONDITION STATEMENT

1. Definition

A traumatic inflammation of the tendon directly below the kneecap (patella), initiated by jumping or climbing activities and resulting in incomplete local tearing of the tendon. Prolonged symptoms are common for many months because of poor blood supply and resulting inflammation.

2. Cause

- Acute, violent jumping episode results in pain below the kneecap (patella) and leads to chronic pain and inflammation.

- Chronic, repetitive jumping, climbing, and running activities can weaken the tendon. Foot imbalance and running up hills are aggravating factors.

3. Subjective Symptoms

- Pain is localized to the tip of the bone just below the kneecap.
- Swelling generally is not present.
- Motion is within normal limits.
- Noise and crepitation usually are not present.
- Giving way is present with hard jumping.

4. Objective Findings

- Tenderness is felt directly on the lower tip of the kneecap.
- Swelling usually is not present.
- Crepitation is not present.
- Instability is not present.

5. Testing Procedures

- X-rays are normal, but a spur may be present in chronic cases.
- Bone scan may be positive at the inferior (lower) pole of the patella.
- In chronic cases, MRI may show an incomplete tear and a chronic tendon problem.
- Arthroscopy is not indicated.

6. Prognosis

Expect many months to a year, in some cases, for complete healing. Some cases never heal, for example, as a result of extreme jumping activities and mountain climbing. Chronic restriction in jumping may be present for 1 to 2 years. Some patients require surgery to remove scarred tendon.

10-POINT TREATMENT PLAN

1. Activity Levels

- Restrict jumping and hard running.

2. Alternative Exercises

- Swimming and biking help to maintain aerobic conditioning.

3. Rehab Exercises

- See rehabilitation exercise program in Part IV of this book.
- Maintain flexibility, endurance, speed, and strength with a patella exercise program.

4. Support

- Neoprene or elastic sports bandages around the patella help reduce the forces on the tendon.
- Orthotics (arch supports) for shoes help to maintain foot control.

5. Thermal Treatment

- Ice after activities to reduce inflammation.
- Heat before activities to maintain muscle flexibility.

6. Medication

- For oral medication, see "The 10-Point Treatment Plan" in Part II of this book.
- A local steroid injection may be helpful, but the tendon should not be injected directly. Frequent injections may further weaken and tear the tendon.

7. Equipment

- Avoid using machines such as bikes and rowing machines that excessively bend the knee.
- Use shoes with excellent pronation control.
- An orthotic (arch support) may be necessary if foot imbalance is present.

8. Nutrition

- Avoid weight gain during periods of inactivity.
- See nutrition suggestions in Part V of this book.

9. Fluids

- Maintain excellent hydration.

10. Surfaces

- Avoid hills and rough surfaces, which torque and stress the patella.

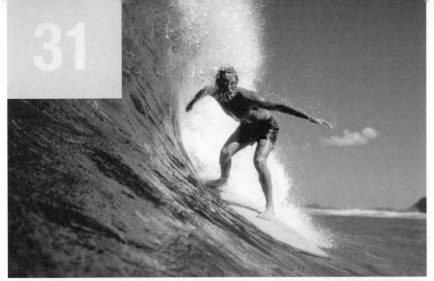

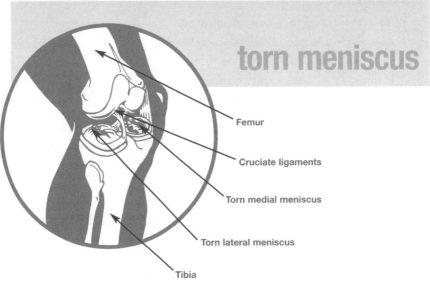

torn meniscus

Femur

Cruciate ligaments

Torn medial meniscus

Torn lateral meniscus

Tibia

6-POINT CONDITION STATEMENT

1. Definition

A traumatic cartilage condition associated with wearing and eventual tearing of the fibrocartilage (the meniscus), the main shock absorber of the knee and the structure that provides cushioning, between the femur and the tibia.

2. Cause

- Acute twisting trauma, such as a hard flexion or rotation injury in skiing or surfing.
- A chronic overuse condition from repetitive bending and frequent twisting.

3. Subjective Symptoms

- Well-localized tenderness on the joint line, leading to progressive pain and swelling.
- Locking of the joint, a feature in some cases.
- Stability is good, but a sensation of giving way is present in some cases.

4. Objective Findings

- Tenderness is well localized at the joint line.
- Limp may be present, especially with bending and twisting.
- Swelling is present.
- Clicking sensation may be felt.

5. Testing Procedures

- Routine x-rays usually are normal.
- Bone scan will show some local inflammation but is not diagnostic.
- MRI is very reliable for subtle tear, but caution is needed for false-positive.
- Arthroscopy should be done if conservative treatment fails.

6. Prognosis

Untreated, the symptoms will subside if activities are greatly reduced. Some cases will heal spontaneously if the tear is in the outer portion of the meniscus near the blood supply. If activity has to be maintained and symptoms persist, arthroscopic surgery should be done to remove the torn portion or repair the meniscus.

10-POINT TREATMENT PLAN

1. Activity Levels

- Let pain be the guide, and avoid any repeated, hard twisting or bending maneuvers.

2. Alternative Exercises

- Avoid activities that require twisting.
- Walking, swimming, biking, and light running are satisfactory if pain is minimal.

3. Rehab Exercises

- See rehabilitation exercise program in Part IV of this book.
- Quadriceps and hamstring strengthening should be done with gentle weight lifting, using free weights or isokinetic machines.
- Let pain be the guide, and do not force exercise.

4. Support

- Bracing can help until muscle development is improved.
- Simple front lace-up brace with metal hinges can help.

5. Thermal Treatment

- Local ice massage helps to relieve symptoms but generally will not correct the mechanical problem.

6. Medication

- For oral medication, see "The 10-Point Treatment Plan" in Part II of this book.
- Local steroid injection sometimes helps to reduce the local synovitis and inflammation.

7. Equipment

- Avoid excessive lateral heel wear in the shoe.
- Use good, firm-heeled shoes.

8. Nutrition

- Avoid weight gain during periods of inactivity.
- See nutrition suggestions in Part V of this book.

9. Fluids

- Maintain excellent hydration.

10. Surfaces

- Avoid any rough surfaces that may twist the knee.
- Do most activities on straight paths.

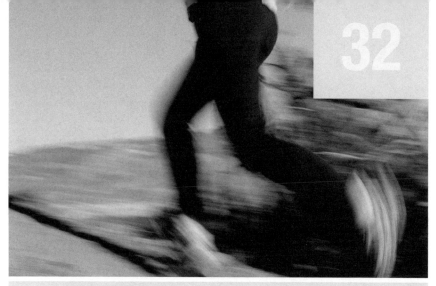

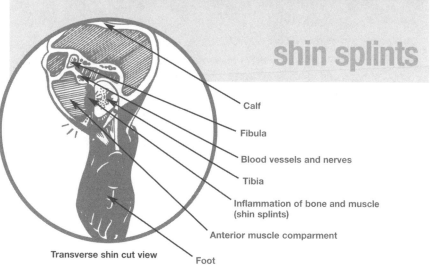

shin splints

Calf

Fibula

Blood vessels and nerves

Tibia

Inflammation of bone and muscle
(shin splints)

Anterior muscle comparment

Transverse shin cut view   Foot

6-POINT CONDITION STATEMENT

1. Definition

An inflammation along the periosteum (outer lining of the bone), characterized by a diffused pain along the front of the shin and due to repetitive stress.

2. Cause

- Associated with a foot imbalance and repetitive running on hard surfaces.
- If prolonged, may progress to a stress fracture.

3. Subjective Symptoms

- Diffused pain along the inner side of the shin starts 2 to 3 inches below the knee and runs to the ankle.

- Thickening of the muscle belly and muscle tenderness can develop.
- Local swelling may be present.
- If swelling increases, nerve symptoms such as numbness and weakness of the foot can develop. This is known as compartment syndrome.

4. Objective Findings

- Diffuse and localized tenderness of the muscle and bone.
- Firmness of the muscle.
- Running with external rotation and a pronated foot.
- Late nerve damage is detected in compartment syndrome in some cases.

5. Testing Procedures

- Routine x-rays usually are normal.
- Compartment testing, involving placement of a needle in the muscle, may show increased muscle pressure.
- MRI is not helpful.
- Bone scan may show diffuse bone inflammation and may help rule out a fracture.

6. Prognosis

Healing usually progresses as you reduce training, correct muscle imbalance, and treat inflammation. If healing is prolonged, a stress fracture can develop.

10-POINT TREATMENT PLAN

1. Activity Levels

- Reduce running or jumping on hard surfaces.

2. Alternative Exercises

- Running in a swimming pool is an excellent aerobic alternative.
- Biking, race walking, and cross-country skiing are excellent alternatives during the pain.

3. Rehab Exercises

- See rehabilitation exercise program in Part IV of this book.

- Rest if injury is very painful, and reduce intensity of aerobic exercise.
- Gradually increase muscle strength and muscle flexibility with weights and rubber tubing.
- Progress to biking and swimming.

4. Support

- Wrap the shins with elastic wraps, or apply taping.
- Neoprene shin guards may be helpful.
- Be careful not to apply too much pressure, which may lead to a compartment syndrome.
- Wear a shoe with a good arch support.

5. Thermal Treatment

- Ice massage to reduce pain and swelling after activity.
- Local heat before activity to relax muscles.

6. Medication

- For oral medication, see "The 10-Point Treatment Plan" in Part II of this book.
- If a local area of pain persists after several months, a local steroid injection may be given.

7. Equipment

- A stabilizing, shock-absorbing shoe.
- An arch support or an orthotic added to the shoe for foot imbalance.

8. Nutrition

- Avoid weight gain during periods of inactivity.
- See nutrition suggestions in Part V of this book.

9. Fluids

- Maintain excellent hydration.

10. Surfaces

- Avoid hills and rough terrain.
- Run on soft surfaces, such as blacktop and bicycle paths.

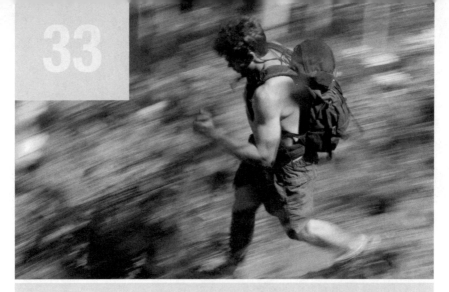

tibia or fibula stress fracture

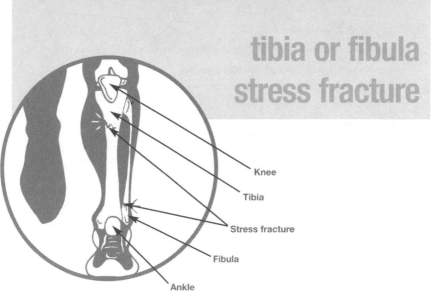

Knee

Tibia

Stress fracture

Fibula

Ankle

6-POINT CONDITION STATEMENT

1. Definition

A traumatic bone condition characterized by early persistent inflammation from shin splints, leading to persistent weakening of the bone and actual crack or fracture.

2. Cause

- Repetitive overuse associated with muscle imbalance and poor alignment of the leg, leading to actual weakening and fracture of the bone.
- Leg malalignment with foot pronation.

- Running in poor shoes on concrete.
- Eating disorder with excess weight loss.

3. Subjective Symptoms

- Initial diffuse pain progresses to a well-localized point of pain, generally on the tibia on the inside of the shin or the outer aspect of the leg above the ankle (fibular bone).
- Vague pain and slight limp can progress to severe local pain and limp.
- Swelling generally is not present until late.
- Nerve symptoms are not present.
- Pain with impact and use is relieved by rest.

4. Objective Findings

- Bone tenderness is well localized.
- Occasionally, local swelling may be present.
- Neurologic exam is normal.

5. Testing Procedures

- Initial x-rays may be normal, but after several weeks a fracture and a healing bone formation may appear.
- Initial bone scan is very helpful in substantiating the diagnosis and in indicating progress by the intensity of the scan.
- MRI may show subtle fracture.

6. Prognosis

With adequate rest, healing generally occurs after 2 to 3 months. Casting generally is not necessary. Displacement of the fracture is very unusual. With a program of rest and gradual walking, swimming, and biking, progressive healing occurs. Long-term treatment with foot correction device such as an orthotic is helpful.

10-POINT TREATMENT PLAN

1. Activity Levels

- Initially, running must be curtailed.
- Avoid any activity that causes a limp or pain.

2. Alternative Exercises

- Running in a swimming pool is an excellent way of maintaining aerobic activity and reducing impact on the bone.
- Race walking, cross-country skiing, and rowing are all permissible if very little pain is produced.

3. Rehab Exercises

- See rehabilitation exercise program in Part IV of this book.
- Inactivity and eliminating impact are key.
- Alternative walking and biking are permissible if pain is minimal.

4. Support

- Wrapping an elastic bandage or Neoprene on the shin may help during early rehabilitation.

5. Thermal Treatment

- Apply ice massage initially, but this should not be a substitute for rest.

6. Medication

- For oral medication, see "The 10-Point Treatment Plan" in Part II of this book.
- Steroid injection is not indicated.
- Overmedication may mask the fracture.
- Calcium tablets and vitamins are not needed unless there is an eating disorder.

7. Equipment

- A good stable, antipronation shoe is very important for prevention.
- An orthotic arch support may be necessary to prevent foot imbalance.

8. Nutrition

- Avoid weight gain during periods of inactivity.
- See nutrition suggestions in Part V of this book.

9. Fluids

- Maintain excellent hydration.

10. Surfaces

- Avoid concrete or hard paths during a running program.
- Avoid hills during the initial healing phase.

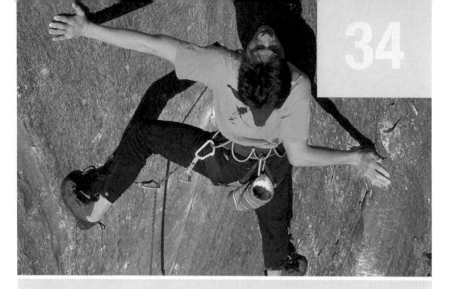

rupture of the gastrocnemius muscle

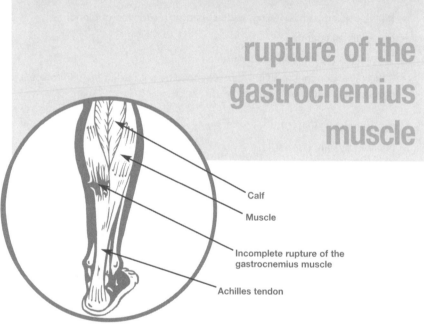

Calf

Muscle

Incomplete rupture of the gastrocnemius muscle

Achilles tendon

Rear view of the calf

6-POINT CONDITION STATEMENT

1. Definition

A traumatic muscle condition, typically seen in a middle-aged athlete and characterized by sudden partial tearing of the inner muscle belly of the calf, generally during a sudden jump, as in rock climbing.

2. Cause

- Sudden, violent jumping or pushing off, causing overloading and tearing of the muscle on the medial (inner) aspect of the muscle belly of the calf.
- Muscle tightness is present generally in a middle-aged male.

3. Subjective Symptoms

- Sudden onset of intense pain, as if you have been kicked or hit by a ball.
- Progressive limping and swelling.
- Symptoms are reduced by using a heel lift.

4. Objective Findings

- Well-localized pain, swelling, and hematoma (collection of blood).
- Nerve usually normal.
- Great difficulty walking on tiptoe.
- Achilles tendon mechanism intact (checked by squeezing the calf to see if it produces a flexion of the foot).

5. Testing Procedures

- Initial x-rays are normal.
- MRI generally is not necessary but could possibly show a small tear of the muscle.
- Bone scan is negative.

6. Prognosis

Generally, 6 to 8 weeks of healing is required. Once healed, the muscle tends to be normal, and recurrences are highly unusual. The main complication could be thrombophlebitis or blood clot formation, due to the swelling and compression of veins. The condition tends to occur in middle-aged people who are developing increasing tightness and weakness. Thrombophlebitis and blood clot formation should be prevented.

10-POINT TREATMENT PLAN

1. Activity Levels

- Early biking, swimming, and walking are satisfactory.

- Lift 5- to 10-pound ankle weights, increasing the weight gradually, to rehabilitate and maintain muscle strength, flexibility, and endurance.

2. Alternative Exercises

- Running in a swimming pool is an excellent way of maintaining aerobic activity.
- Gentle biking with toe clips balances the force on the front and back of the thigh.

3. Rehab Exercises

- See rehabilitation exercise program in Part IV of this book.
- Rest is indicated during the first several weeks.
- Gentle biking, swimming, and walking can be done, especially with a heel lift.

4. Support

- Add a heel lift.
- Wrap your ankle up to the calf with a light elastic bandage, but not too tight: Too tight a wrap may bring on phlebitis.

5. Thermal Treatment

- Local ice massage will reduce pain and swelling.
- If muscle spasm is severe, local heat can be used.

6. Medication

- For oral medication, see "The 10-Point Treatment Plan" in Part II of this book.
- If after several months a local area of pain persists due to tendinitis, a local steroid injection could be done.

7. Equipment

- Add a 1-inch heel lift to your shoe.
- A cane or crutch may be necessary—consider using a walking pole (see information in Part V).

8. Nutrition

- Avoid weight gain during periods of inactivity.
- See nutrition suggestions in Part V of this book.

9. Fluids

- Maintain excellent hydration.

10. Surfaces

- Avoid running up hills.
- Stay on soft surfaces, such as blacktop and bicycle paths.

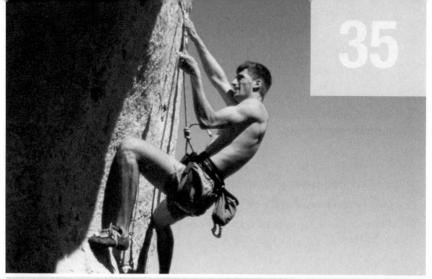

achilles
tendinitis

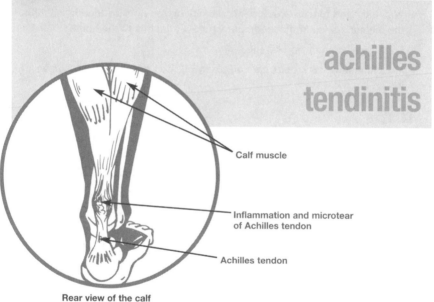

Calf muscle

Inflammation and microtear
of Achilles tendon

Achilles tendon

Rear view of the calf

6-POINT CONDITION STATEMENT

1. Definition

A traumatic or degenerative tendon condition characterized by chronic pain and
inflammation on the back of the ankle along the Achilles tendon, at the junction
where the large muscle group of calf attaches to the heel bone. Not a complete
tear, but a partial tendon fiber disruption and inflammation.

2. Cause

• Acute, sudden jumping or running, causing a microscopic tearing of the
muscle group, possibly in a previously weakened tendon.

- Chronic repetitive microtrauma to Achilles tendon, usually associated with muscle imbalance, excessive running up hills, or both. Foot imbalance is present in some cases.

3. Subjective Symptoms

- Localized pain appears behind the ankle along the Achilles tendon.
- Localized thickening and swelling of the tendon may be present.
- Stiffness: The ankle may be tight, and pain may be aggravated by walking on the toes.

4. Objective Findings

- Well-localized tenderness appears directly on the Achilles tendon, either in the midsubstance of the tendon or where it attaches to the bone.
- Local swelling may be present.
- Muscle testing will induce pain on plantar flexion of the ankle and on walking on the toes.

5. Testing Procedures

- Routine x-rays generally are negative, but a small spur on the back of the heel may be present.
- Bone scan is not helpful but may show slight bone inflammation.
- MRI test may show tearing of the tendon in acute and chronic stages.

6. Prognosis

Healing can be prolonged because of poor circulation in the tendon. On a conservative program, slow but progressive healing may occur with incomplete or microchronic tears. If pain persists, open surgical removal of scar tissue in the tendon may be necessary. For acute tears, either casting or surgical treatment is indicated, depending on the activity level of the individual and the philosophy of the surgeon.

10-POINT TREATMENT PLAN

1. Activity Levels

- Proceed with caution. Let pain be the guide.
- Slow, gentle, light running is permissible; try to avoid excessive jumping or propulsion exercises.

2. Alternative Exercises

- Avoid hard jumping and twisting.
- Choose slow, gentle, straight activities, such as race walking.
- Biking and swimming are satisfactory.

3. Rehab Exercises

- See rehabilitation exercise program in Part IV of this book.
- Do strengthening exercises for the front muscles of the shin and gentle stretching exercises for the calf muscle.

4. Support

- Wrap the Achilles area and the calf with an elastic bandage or tape.
- The main support is a proper shoe with a stable heel.

5. Thermal Treatment

- Local ice massage to reduce inflammation.
- Heat before and after activity to loosen muscles.

6. Medication

- For oral medication, see "The 10-Point Treatment Plan" in Part II of this book.
- Local steroid injection is sometimes indicated in the tendon sheath, but not directly into the tendon.

7. Equipment

- A very stable running shoe with an elevated heel to reduce the pressure on the heel.
- Simple orthotics (arch supports) in the shoe to control pronation. Custom-made orthotics are helpful in some cases.

8. Nutrition

- Avoid weight gain during periods of inactivity.
- See nutrition suggestions in Part V of this book.

9. Fluids

- Maintain excellent hydration.

10. Surfaces

- Avoid steep inclines and hills.
- Stay on soft surfaces, such as blacktop and asphalt biking paths.

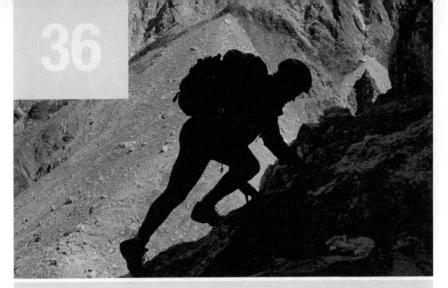

36

torn achilles tendon

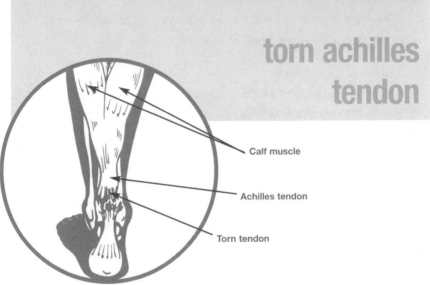

Calf muscle

Achilles tendon

Torn tendon

Rear view of the calf

6-POINT CONDITION STATEMENT

1. Definition

A traumatic tendon condition characterized by a total disruption of the large tendon behind the ankle (Achilles tendon), resulting in acute pain and inability to walk.

2. Cause

- A slow, gradual deterioration or degeneration of the tendon.
- An acute, sudden overload, causing total disruption of the fibers.

- In a middle-aged person, an overloading on the Achilles tendon; possibly also associated with foot imbalance.

3. Subjective Symptoms

- Gradual pain behind the ankle, leading to exposure and intensive pain and a sharp sensation, as if you were kicked or hit.
- Total inability to walk on the toes.
- Progressive swelling.

4. Objective Findings

- There is well-localized tenderness and a gap in the Achilles tendon.
- Squeezing the calf (Thompson's test) produces no plantar flexion of the ankle.
- Neurologic exam is normal.

5. Testing Procedures

- Routine x-rays are negative, but a small spur may appear.
- Degenerative changes may be present in the bone.
- Arthrogram is not helpful.
- MRI may show disruption of the tendon.

6. Prognosis

Many philosophies of treatment are available. Some surgeons recommend immediate surgery. Some recommend casting for 2 to 3 months. Six to 9 months of healing may be required before returning to jumping activities. This injury may threaten careers in sports that require jumping, such as rock climbing and mountaineering.

10-POINT TREATMENT PLAN

1. Activity Levels

- During casting, biking with the well leg, walking, and upper-body aerobic conditioning and weight lifting are indicated.

2. Alternative Exercises

- Running in a swimming pool, with a plastic bag over the cast.

- Biking with the well leg.
- Upper-body rowing.

3. Rehab Exercises

- See rehabilitation exercise program in Part IV of this book.
- Do upper-body exercises during casting.

4. Support

- Cast is indicated for many months, followed by an air-bag ankle splint.
- Progress to simple elastic ankle wraps and a heel lift.

5. Thermal Treatment

- Ice massage initially to reduce pain and swelling.
- Local heat to the calf to reduce muscle soreness.

6. Medication

- For oral medication, see "The 10-Point Treatment Plan" in Part II of this book.
- Avoid steroid injections.

7. Equipment

- Initially, a cast is required with the foot in plantar flexion (toes down), whether or not your have surgery.
- Use aerodyne bike for upper-body exercise.

8. Nutrition

- Avoid weight gain during periods of inactivity.
- See nutrition suggestions in Part V of this book.

9. Fluids

- Maintain excellent hydration.

10. Surfaces

- Avoid exercising on hills and performing twisting activities.
- When cast is removed and rehabilitation has progressed appropriately, run on soft surfaces, such as blacktop and bicycle paths.

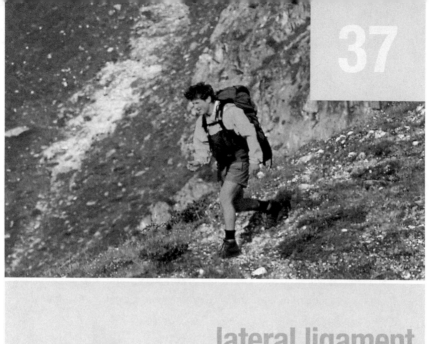

lateral ligament sprain

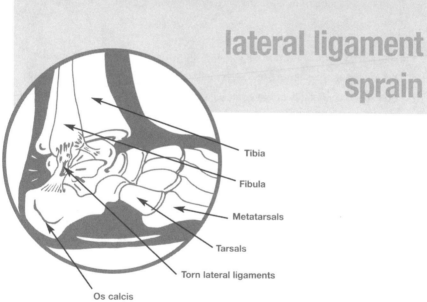

Tibia

Fibula

Metatarsals

Tarsals

Torn lateral ligaments

Os calcis

6-POINT CONDITION STATEMENT

1. Definition

   A traumatic ankle injury, associated with a twisting injury to the outer (lateral) ligaments; associated with acute pain, swelling, and limp.

2. Cause

   - Acute: a sudden twisting or inversion (an inward tilting) of the ankle.
   - Chronic: repetitive ankle sprains with progressive stretching and tearing of the ligaments; may lead to chronic recurrent instability.

3. Subjective Symptoms

- Pain is well localized to the outer tip of the ankle bone.
- Swelling occurs within a few hours.
- A sensation of giving way is present with repeated sprains.
- Crepitation generally is not present.

4. Objective Findings

- Tenderness is well localized to the outer tip of the ankle bone.
- Swelling is present from local bleeding.
- Instability: Ligament testing will reveal the ankle is giving way.
- Stiffness and loss of motion are present because of swelling and pain.

5. Testing Procedures

- Initial x-rays are usually normal but may show associated small fractures.
- Chronic cases may show bone spurs and loose fragments on stress x-rays.
- Bone scan generally is not indicated.
- MRI may show ligament tearing.
- Arthroscopy generally is not indicated but may reveal bony fragments in chronic cases.

6. Prognosis

With proper treatment, rest, and rehabilitation, acute cases usually heal with a resulting stable ankle. Chronic, recurrent tears in a loose-jointed person may lead to a chronically unstable ankle, which may require surgical reconstruction of the ligaments.

10-POINT TREATMENT PLAN

1. Activity Levels

- During initial splinting and casting, let pain be the guide.
- Maintain general aerobic conditioning and upper-body strength.

2. Alternative Exercises

- Swimming and running in a pool may be advisable with the permission of a physician.

- A plastic bag can be put over the ankle if a cast is used.
- Upper-body aerobic conditioning and weight lifting are permissible.

3. Rehab Exercises

- See rehabilitation exercise program in Part IV of this book.
- During casting, continue isometric ankle and knee exercises.
- During rehabilitation, work on flexibility and strength with weights and tubing.

4. Support

- Acute cases may need tape, splints, or a cast.
- Chronic cases during rehabilitation may need air stirrup splints.

5. Thermal Treatment

- Apply ice locally for the first 2 or 3 days.
- Avoid heat if any unusual swelling is present.

6. Medication

- For oral medication, see "The 10-Point Treatment Plan" in Part II of this book.

7. Equipment

- Wear high-top shoes with extremely stable heels.

8. Nutrition

- Avoid weight gain during periods of inactivity.
- See nutrition suggestions in Part V of this book.

9. Fluids

- Maintain excellent hydration.

10. Surfaces

- Be very cautious when running on uneven ground and terrain.
- Avoid running on extremely firm surfaces such as cement.

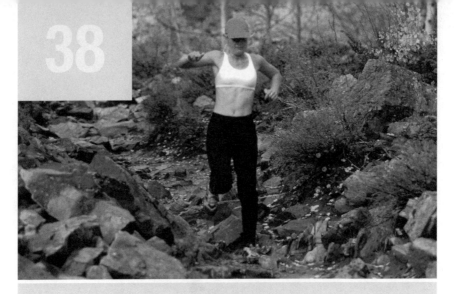

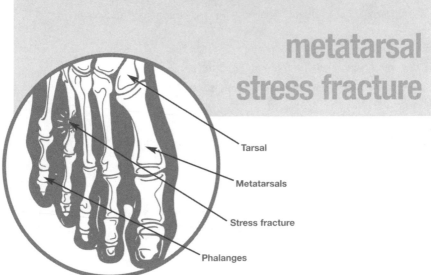

metatarsal stress fracture

Tarsal

Metatarsals

Stress fracture

Phalanges

6-POINT CONDITION STATEMENT

1. Definition

An overuse condition in the bone, characterized by a microfracture of the metatarsal bone. An aching pain in the foot is felt during long-distance running.

2. Cause

- Acute: a sudden pain or snap in a previously weakened bone; occurs during a jump.
- Chronic: repeated microtrauma in a runner with foot imbalance who performs on hard surfaces. Associated factors: obesity, malnutrition, and, in some cases, eating disorders.

3. Subjective Symptoms

- Pain is well localized directly over the bone on the top of the foot.
- Swelling initially is not present.
- Stiffness is present after running.
- Crepitation is not present.

4. Objective Findings

- Tenderness is well localized to the bone surface.
- Local swelling may be present as the healing bone forms.
- Loss of motion is not present.

5. Testing Procedures

- Initial x-rays may be normal, but x-rays 2 or 3 weeks later will show healing bone formation.
- Bone scan will be very diagnostic.
- MRI is not required.

6. Prognosis

The most important aspect of this condition is proper recognition and diagnosis; otherwise, many months of bone healing will be required. Total rest is not required. Casting generally is not needed. Many alternatives are available. Proper shoes and orthotics are very helpful. Avoiding obesity and malnutrition is important.

10-POINT TREATMENT PLAN

1. Activity Levels

- Reducing intensity of outdoor recreation is important, but there is no need to stop all activities. Let pain be the guide.
- Displacement of the fracture is unusual with moderate activity.

2. Alternative Exercises

- Running in water, biking, and swimming are acceptable.

3. Rehab Exercises

- See rehabilitation exercise program in Part IV of this book.

- Maintain flexibility, endurance, speed, and strength of the muscles and joints above and below the fracture.

4. Support

- Casting is rarely indicated, unless pain and swelling are severe.
- Simple protective activities and a good supporting shoe are enough to protect the bone.

5. Thermal Treatment

- Ice massage helps to reduce pain and swelling.

6. Medication

- For oral medication, see "The 10-Point Treatment Plan" in Part II of this book.
- Avoid medications that may mask the pain and prevent a proper diagnosis.
- Calcium and vitamins are suggested if an eating disorder is present.

7. Equipment

- Proper shoes with good heel control.
- Orthotics (arch supports) for pronated feet.

8. Nutrition

- Avoid weight gain during periods of inactivity.
- See nutrition suggestions in Part V of this book.

9. Fluids

- Maintain excellent hydration.

10. Surfaces

- It is very important to avoid running on concrete or any rough surfaces that cause excessive impact to the foot.

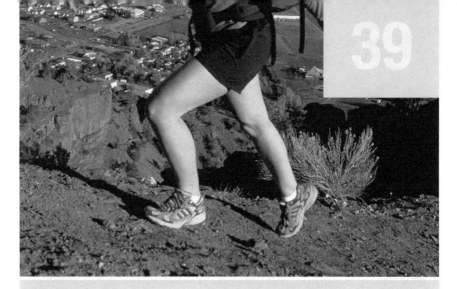

morton's
neuroma

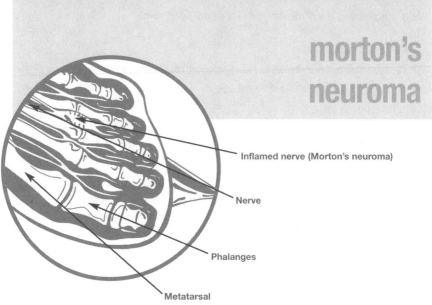

Inflamed nerve (Morton's neuroma)

Nerve

Phalanges

Metatarsal

6-POINT CONDITION STATEMENT

1. Definition

A traumatic nerve compression of the foot characterized by numbness of the third and fourth toes; associated with tight shoes and pronated foot (weak arches).

2. Cause

- Acute: direct injury to the top of the foot, with resulting swelling and compression of the nerve.

- Chronic: microtrauma to the nerve between the third and fourth toes; may result in a "Morton's foot" (a short first toe and a pronated foot).

3. Subjective Symptoms

- Pain between the third and fourth toes, radiating to the foot.
- Swelling generally is not present.
- Limp is present when individual wears tight high-heeled shoes.

4. Objective Findings

- Tenderness is well localized in the web between the third and fourth toes.
- Pinching the nerve produces numbness.
- Compressing the forefoot reproduces the symptoms.

5. Testing Procedures

- X-rays usually are normal, but a shortened first toe may be noted.
- Bone scan generally is not necessary.
- MRI is not helpful.
- EMG generally is not necessary.

6. Prognosis

Relief is usual with conservative treatment: orthotics, rest, and possibly a local steroid injection. Surgery to excise the nerve may be necessary in chronic cases. Following surgery, the patient usually has relief from pain but may always feel numbness in the toes.

10-POINT TREATMENT PLAN

1. Activity Levels

- Continue activities such as running and biking, but with moderation.

2. Alternative Exercises

- Stress upper-body weight lifting and biking.

3. Rehab Exercises

- See rehabilitation exercise program in Part IV of this book.

- Let pain be the guide.
- Reduce intensity of running and biking, but there is no need to stop.

4. Support

- A metatarsal bar on the shoe and an orthotic for the arch are helpful.

5. Thermal Treatment

- Local ice massage to reduce pain and swelling

6. Medication

- For oral medication, see "The 10-Point Treatment Plan" in Part II of this book.
- Local steroid injection around the nerve may be helpful.

7. Equipment

- Shoes should be wide and have ample room for the toes.
- Be careful of tight toe clips on bicycles.

8. Nutrition

- Avoid weight gain during periods of inactivity.
- See nutrition suggestions in Part V of this book.

9. Fluids

- Maintain excellent hydration.

10. Surfaces

- Beware of hard impact on rough surfaces and concrete.

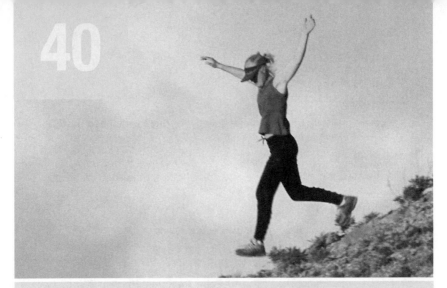

plantar fasciitis (heel pain)

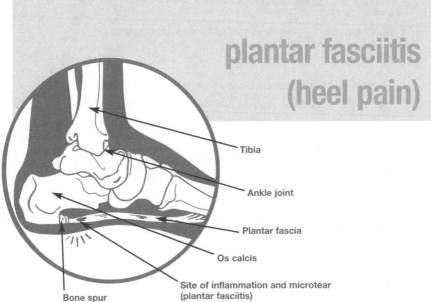

Tibia

Ankle joint

Plantar fascia

Os calcis

Site of inflammation and microtear
(plantar fasciitis)

Bone spur

6-POINT CONDITION STATEMENT

1. Definition

A traumatic, degenerative process characterized by pain along the inner aspect of the heel and radiating along the arch; may occur in a young runner or a middle-aged worker with foot imbalance.

2. Cause

- Acute: violent jumping and tearing of the plantar fascia (the heavy ligament band along the arch).

- Chronic: microtrauma or overuse of the foot; associated with foot imbalance, muscle imbalance, and tight ligaments in the foot.

3. Subjective Symptoms

- Pain, especially on awakening in the morning and with first steps.
- Swelling generally is not present.
- Stiffness is present, especially in the morning, when weight bears down on the rested foot.
- Occasional numbness in the heel.

4. Objective Findings

- Tenderness is well localized to the inner aspect of the heel.
- Swelling generally is not present.
- Instability of the foot may be present with a pronated foot.
- Nerve exam is usually normal.

5. Testing Procedures

- X-rays may be normal, but a spur on the heel may be present.
- Scan may show a positive area on the bone where the ligament attaches.
- MRI generally is not necessary.
- Arthroscopy is not done.

6. Prognosis

Chronic pain due to poor healing is usual because of poor circulation to the ligament and stresses to the heel. Referral to a sports podiatrist to fabricate orthotics may be necessary. Surgery is unusual, but with chronic cases, the injury may require cutting the ligament where it attaches to the heel.

10-POINT TREATMENT PLAN

1. Activity Levels

- Continue with moderate running, biking, and jumping, but avoid extremes.

2. Alternative Exercises

- Biking and swimming are excellent alternatives during rehabilitation.

3. Rehab Exercises

- See rehabilitation exercise program in Part IV of this book.
- Maintain foot flexibility and strength with tubing and simple weights.

4. Support

- Orthotic device in the shoe to support the arch is helpful.

5. Thermal Treatment

- Local ice massage to the painful area.
- Heat to relieve muscle spasm and tightness.

6. Medication

- For oral medication, see "The 10-Point Treatment Plan" in Part II of this book.
- Local injection of steroid may be helpful in chronic cases.

7. Equipment

- Use a good, firm-heeled shoe that supports the arch.

8. Nutrition

- Avoid weight gain during periods of inactivity.
- See nutrition suggestions in Part V of this book.

9. Fluids

- Maintain excellent hydration.

10. Surfaces

- Avoid excessive running on hard surfaces such as concrete.
- Avoid running on curves.

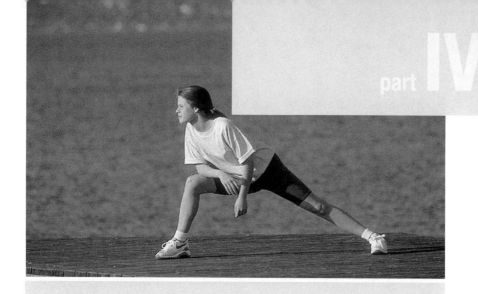

rehabilitation exercise programs

by Erin Doxtator, MPT, LAT

Even in physical therapy, it is important to listen to your body. Some patients experience an aggravation of their basic injury because the exercise program is too aggressive. The programs outlined in this section offer you a graduated and moderate program of rehabilitation to regain your strength and flexibility without reinjury.

The following section outlines thirteen specific exercise programs that I commonly use with my patients at the Performance Centers of St. Francis Hospital in Milwaukee to build strength and flexibility following injury, and to help prevent reinjury upon return to their outdoor activities.

These exercise programs fall into two categories: strengthening and stretching. Some of the strengthening exercises require that resistance be used in the form of resistive bands or wraparound weights. These can be purchased at sporting goods stores.

Stretching exercises can be performed both before and after activity. Stretching exercises are most effective when the muscles being stretched are already warm. This means warming up the muscles by performing a lighter version of the activity you are to perform (hiking, biking) for 5 to 10 minutes, then perform your stretching exercises. Stretching after activity is very effective because the muscles are thoroughly warmed up and very accepting of stretch. It is important that you do not overstretch muscles because injuries can occur. When stretching a muscle, pull only until a gentle stretch is felt in the muscle, and never bounce. If you are feeling pain when you stretch, it is an indication that you are pulling too hard and possibly causing injury. A muscle will become more flexible with gentle stretches of longer duration, 20 to 30 seconds.

It is important to remember that spending a little time away from your favorite outdoor activities strengthening and stretching is very important in preventing injuries from occurring. Keeping yourself strong and flexible, as well as avoiding repetitive bending and twisting activities, will help keep you going in your outdoor activities year-round.

- Upper Extremity Stretching Program..181
- Lower Extremity Stretching Program...182
- Back Strengthening Program...184
- Beginning Shoulder Program..187
- Rotator Cuff Program 190
- Shoulder Acromioclavicular Program 194
- Shoulder Dislocation Program 197
- Lateral Epicondylitis Program—Beginning..200
- Lateral Epicondylitis Program—Advanced..202
- Patellar Program 204
- Meniscus Program..206
- Anterior Cruciate Ligament (ACL) Program...208
- Ankle Program 210

These same exercises are used by physicians, physical therapists, and athletic trainers at Covenant Rehabilitation Services of Milwaukee for rehabilitation purposes following injury. Before starting any exercise program, especially following an injury, it is important that you consult a physician. The physician can help you decide which exercises are appropriate, as well as the number of sets and repetitions and whether or not you need to add weight to your exercises. If the physician feels you need more guidance with an exercise program, he or she may refer you to a physical therapist, who will guide you through your program.

Erin Doxtator, MPT, LAT, is a physical therapist and athletic trainer at the Performance Centers of St. Francis Hospital in Milwaukee. She received her bachelor of science degree in exercise science from the University of Wisconsin and a master's degree in physical therapy from Northwestern University. She is an avid bicyclist.

Upper Extremity Stretching Program

Stretching or flexibility exercises are performed to lengthen the muscle, thereby increasing the efficiency of the muscle and reducing the incidence of muscle strain, pulls, and tears. To maximize the effectiveness of your stretching routine: (1) DO NOT BOUNCE. (2) Hold the stretch for 20 to 30 seconds. (3) Repeat each stretch 3 to 5 times. Keep in mind that stretching should be slightly uncomfortable but not painful. For best results, perform these stretching exercises after muscles have been slightly warmed up. These stretches should also be incorporated into your normal cool-down routine.

1. ANTERIOR SHOULDER STRETCH

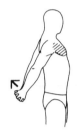

- Interlock fingers behind your back, with elbows turned in and arms straight.
- Lift arms up until you feel a stretch in your shoulders and chest.

2. POSTERIOR SHOULDER/ SIDE STRETCH

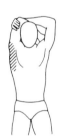

- With arm to be stretched, reach over opposite shoulder, keeping arm behind head.
- Gently pull elbow behind head with opposite arm.

Variation: In same position, bend from your hips away from the shoulder to be stretched.

3. POSTERIOR SHOULDER STRETCH

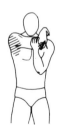

- Reach arm to be stretched across front of chest.
- Grasp elbow or arm to be stretched with opposite hand.
- Apply light pressure to elbow, moving arm closer to chest.

4. INTERNAL ROTATOR STRETCH

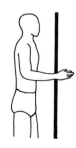

- With elbow bent at 90 degrees, place palm of arm to be stretched against edge of wall or immovable object.
- While maintaining this position, gradually twist away from arm toward opposite shoulder.
- Do not push hand against wall.

5. WRIST FLEXOR STRETCH

- With elbow straight, raise arm up in front of you to shoulder height with palm up.

- Bend wrist down and grasp hand with opposite hand.

- Pull back gently until a stretch is felt on the bottom of the forearm.

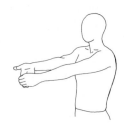

6. WRIST EXTENSOR STRETCH

- With elbow straight, raise arm up in front of you to shoulder height with palm down.

- Bend wrist down and grasp hand with opposite hand.

- Pull back gently until a stretch is felt on the top of the forearm.

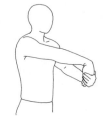

Lower Extremity Stretching Program

1. ILIOTIBIAL (IT) BAND STRETCHING (SITTING)

- Sit on the floor with leg to be stretched crossed over opposite leg. Support self with arm outstretched behind you.

- Pull leg to be stretched with opposite arm toward opposite shoulder until a stretch is felt on the outside part of the hip.

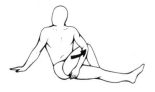

2. HAMSTRING STRETCH (SITTING)

- Sit on the floor with leg to be stretched extended out in front of you.

- Bend opposite leg so that bottom of foot is resting against thigh of straight leg.

- Slowly bend forward at the hips, keeping your back straight until a stretch is felt behind the knee and thigh. Be sure not to bend knee of leg being stretched.

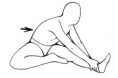

3. INNER THIGH (GROIN)

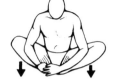

- Sit on the floor with knees bent and soles of feet facing each other.

- Slowly push down on inner thighs with forearms until a gentle stretch is felt.

4. KNEES TO CHEST

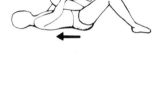

- Lie down on your back.

- Using your arms, bring left knee up toward chest until a stretch is felt in your lower back.

- Repeat with right leg.

5. QUAD STRETCH

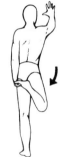

- While standing, support yourself against a wall or chair.

- Extend leg to be stretched behind you, bend your knee and hold the foot of the leg to be stretched with your opposite hand, gently pulling your heel toward your buttocks until a stretch is felt in the front of the thigh.

6. GASTROCNEMIUS AND SOLEUS STRETCH

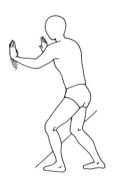

- Face a wall and stand about 2 feet away. Place palms flat against the wall, and step forward with one foot, placing the leg to be stretched straight behind you.

- Bend opposite leg and place foot flat on the floor in front of you.

- Keep heel of back leg down and slowly move your hips forward toward the wall, keeping your back straight until a stretch is felt in the calf.

- Repeat the exercise with back leg slightly bent at the knee.

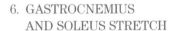

7. ILIOTIBIAL (IT) BAND STRETCH (STANDING)

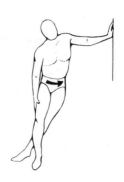

- Stand with side to be stretched facing the wall, arm's-length away. Place hand on wall for support.
- Cross opposite leg over leg to be stretched and slowly lean hip into wall until a stretch is felt on the outside part of the hip.

Back Strengthening Program

The following exercises are designed to help strengthen the extensor muscles of your thoracic and lumbar spine. If you have increased pain with any of the exercises, please let your therapist know.

1. PRONE ON ELBOWS

- Lie down on your stomach.
- Prop yourself up on your elbows, allowing your lower back to sag.
- Hold for 10 seconds. Relax.
- Perform ___ sets, ___ repetitions, ___ times/day.

2. PRONE PRESS-UPS

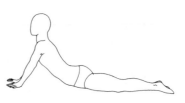

- Lie down on your stomach.
- Place hands at shoulder level as if you were going to do a push-up.
- Press up by straightening your elbows, allowing your hips to remain on the floor and your lower back to extend.
- Hold for ___ seconds. Relax.
- Perform ___ sets, ___ repetitions, ___ times/day.

3. ARM LIFTS

- Lie down on your stomach with arms above head and legs straight.
- Raise one arm 3 to 6 inches off floor.
- Hold for 5 seconds. Relax.
- Repeat with other arm.
- Perform ___ sets, ___ repetitions, ___ times/day.

4. LEG LIFTS

- Lie down on your stomach with legs straight.
- Raise one leg 3 to 6 inches off floor.
- Hold for 5 seconds. Relax.
- Repeat with other leg.
- Perform ___ sets, ___ repetitions, ___ times/day.

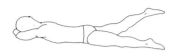

5. ALTERNATE ARM AND LEG LIFTS

- Lie down on your stomach with arms above head and legs straight.
- Raise left arm and right leg simultaneously 3 to 6 inches off floor.
- Hold for 5 seconds. Relax.
- Repeat with right arm and left leg.
- Perform ___ sets, ___ repetitions, ___ times/day.

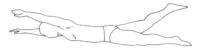

6. BILATERAL ARM LIFTS

- Lie down on your stomach with arms above head and legs straight.
- Raise both arms 3 to 6 inches off the floor at the same time.
- Hold for 5 seconds. Relax.
- Perform ___ sets, ___ repetitions, ___ times/day.

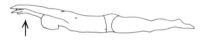

7. CHEST LIFTS

- Lie down on your stomach with a pillow under hips. Arms should be at sides and legs straight.
- Raise upper body off floor to a horizontal position.
- Hold for 5 seconds. Relax.
- Perform ___ sets, ___ repetitions, ___ times/day.

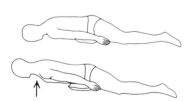

8. BRIDGING

- Lie down on your back with knees bent up and feet flat on floor.
- Raise buttocks off floor until level with knees.
- Hold for 5 seconds. Relax.
- Perform ___ sets, ___ repetitions, ___ times/day.

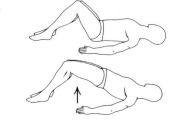

9. 4-POINT ALTERNATE ARM AND LEG LIFTS

- Assume hands-and-knees position.
- Raise left arm and right leg off floor to horizontal position simultaneously.
- Hold for 5 seconds. Relax.
- Repeat with right arm and left leg.
- Perform ___ sets, ___ repetitions, ___ times/day.

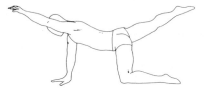

10. CAT/CAMEL

- Assume hands-and-knees position.
- Drop chin and arch back up like a cat.
- Hold for 5 seconds.
- Relax by lifting head and allowing back to sag in the middle like a camel.
- Hold for 5 seconds.
- Perform ___ sets, ___ repetitions, ___ times/day.

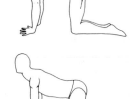

Beginning Shoulder Program

The following exercises are designed for early motion of the shoulder joint in order to prevent scarring and tightening of the joint capsule.

1. CODMAN'S

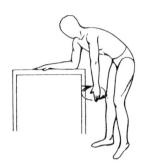

- Support your uninvolved arm on a table or countertop and allow your involved arm to hang freely.

- Keep your elbow straight and initiate a pendular swinging motion using your body.

- Move your arm:
  (a) circles clockwise and counterclockwise.
  (b) side to side.

- Perform ___ sets, ___ repetitions, ___ times/day.

2. CANE EXERCISES

ABDUCTION

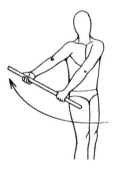

- Stand upright with cane in both hands, with palm of involved arm facing upward.

- Using your uninvolved arm to assist, push cane out to the side and up toward shoulder as far as possible.

- Return to starting position.

- Perform ___ sets, ___ repetitions, ___ times/day.

FLEXION

- Lie on your back with a pillow under your knees and cane held in both hands.

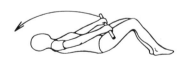

- Keeping your elbows straight, lift cane up over your head as far as possible.

- Return to starting position.

- Perform ___ sets, ___ repetitions, ___ times/day.

HORIZONTAL ABDUCTION

- Lie on your back holding the cane in both hands.
- Lift the cane up to 90 degrees.
- Keeping your elbows straight, move the cane to one side as far as possible, then move the cane to the other side as far as possible.
- Perform ___ sets, ___ repetitions, ___ times/day.

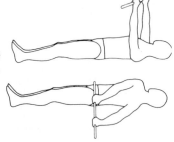

3. INTERNAL/EXTERNAL ROTATION

- Lie on your back with your involved arm lifted up to the side to a comfortable level.
- Rotate your shoulder outward (away from your body) as far as possible, then inward (toward your body) as far as possible.
- Progress to bringing your shoulder out at a 90 degree angle.
- Perform ___ sets, ___ repetitions, ___ times/day.

4. ISOMETRICS

FLEXION

- Stand close to and facing a wall with your involved arm at your side.
- Keeping your elbow straight, push your arm forward into the wall.
- Hold for 5 seconds. Relax.
- Perform ___ sets, ___ repetitions, ___ times/day.

ABDUCTION

- Stand with your involved side facing a wall, with your arm at your side.
- Keeping your elbow straight, push your arm out to the side against the wall.
- Hold for 5 seconds. Relax.
- Perform ___ sets, ___ repetitions, ___ times/day.

EXTENSION

- Stand with your back up against a wall, with your involved arm at your side.
- Keeping your elbow straight, push your arm backward against the wall.
- Hold for 5 seconds. Relax.
- Perform ___ sets, ___ repetitions, ___ times/day.

INTERNAL ROTATION

- Stand with the inside of your involved arm against a wall corner or door frame with your elbow bent to 90 degrees.
- Pull your arm inward against the wall.
- Hold for 5 seconds. Relax.
- Perform ___ sets, ___ repetitions, ___ times/day.

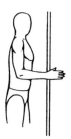

EXTERNAL ROTATION

- Stand with the outside of your involved arm against a wall corner or door frame with your elbow bent to 90 degrees.
- Push your arm outward against the wall.
- Hold for 5 seconds. Relax.
- Perform ___ sets, ___ repetitions, ___ times/day.

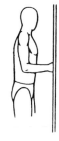

5. SHOULDER SHRUGS

- Sit or stand with your shoulders back and arms at sides.
- Place weight over top of shoulder or in hand.
- Slowly lift (shrug) shoulder up to ears.
- Hold for 5 seconds. Relax.
- Perform ___ sets, ___ repetitions, ___ times/day.

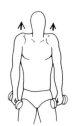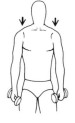

6. SHOULDER RETRACTION

- Rest arms on table at shoulder level.
- Pull arms back as far as possible, pinching shoulder blades together.
- Perform ___ sets, ___ repetitions, ___ times/day.

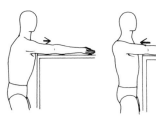

Rotator Cuff Program

The rotator cuff is a group of major shoulder muscles that work together to move the shoulder joint. Rotator cuff injuries can occur with repetitive overhead activities that stretch and impinge the cuff. The following exercises are recommended for strengthening the rotator cuff in order to return to normal activities.

1. INTERNAL ROTATION

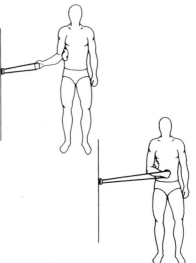

- Place tubing in door at elbow level.
- Stand with your involved side toward the door.
- Bend elbow to 90 degrees and place a towel roll between arm and side.
- Hold tubing in hand and rotate shoulder inward toward opposite hip.
- Return slowly to starting position.
- Perform ___ sets, ___ repetitions, ___ times/day.

2. EXTERNAL ROTATION

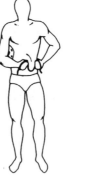
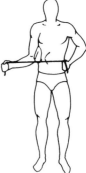

- Wrap tubing around both hands
- Bend elbow of involved arm to 90 degrees and place a towel roll between arm and side.
- Anchor hand of uninvolved shoulder on hip.
- Hold tubing in hand and rotate shoulder outward away from your body.
- Return slowly to starting position.
- Perform ___ sets, ___ repetitions, ___ times/day.

3. EXTENSION IN STANDING

- Place tubing in door at elbow level.
- Face the door, hold tubing in hand of involved side, and pull it straight back behind you, keeping your elbow straight.
- Return slowly to starting position.
- Perform ___ sets, ___ repetitions, ___ times/day.

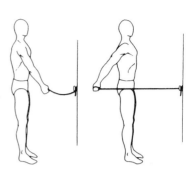

4. FLEXION

- Stand with one end of tubing under the foot of involved side.
- Hold tubing with thumb on top and lift arm straight up in front of you, keeping elbow straight.
- Return slowly to starting position.
- Perform ___ sets, ___ repetitions, ___ times/day.

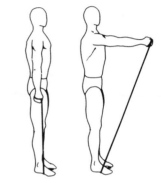

5. ABDUCTION

- Stand with one end of tubing under the foot of involved side.
- Hold tubing with thumb on top and lift arm directly out to the side, keeping elbow straight.
- Return slowly to starting position.
- Perform ___ sets, ___ repetitions, ___ times/day.

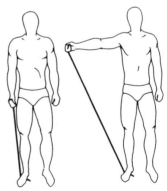

6. EMPTY CAN

- Stand with middle of tubing under your feet.
- Hold tubing in both hands, with thumbs turned down.
- Lift your arms up at a 30-degree forward angle, keeping elbows straight.
- Do not lift above shoulder level.
- Return slowly to starting position.
- Perform ___ sets, ___ repetitions, ___ times/day.

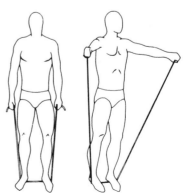

7. HORIZONTAL PULL

- Hold tubing in both hands at shoulder height.
- Pull tubing apart, bringing arms out to each side of your body.
- Return slowly to starting position.
- Perform ___ sets, ___ repetitions, ___ times/day.

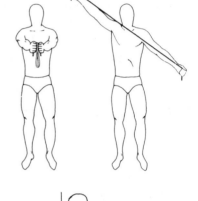

8. DIAGONAL PULL

- Hold tubing in both hands at shoulder height.
- Pull tubing apart at a diagonal, with involved arm moving upward and uninvolved arm moving downward.
- Return slowly to starting position.
- Perform ___ sets, ___ repetitions, ___ times/day.

9. WALL PUSH-UPS

- Stand about 2 feet away from the wall.
- Place hands on wall with fingers pointing in toward each other.
- Slowly bend your elbows, bringing your chest in toward the wall.
- Return slowly to starting position.
- Perform ___ sets, ___ repetitions, ___ times/day.

10. EXTENSION IN LYING

- Lie on your stomach, with your involved arm hanging over the side of bed.
- Tie tubing at hand level to object in front of you.
- Hold tubing and pull arm back and up toward ceiling, keeping elbow straight.
- Return slowly to starting position.
- Perform ___ sets, ___ repetitions, ___ times/day.

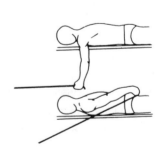

11. HORIZONTAL ABDUCTION

- Lie on your stomach, with your involved arm over the side of bed.
- Tie tubing below shoulder level to stationary object.
- Hold tubing in hand and pull straight out to the side, maintaining shoulder at 90 degrees.
- Return slowly to starting position.
- Perform ___ sets, ___ repetitions, ___ times/day.

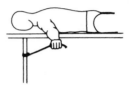
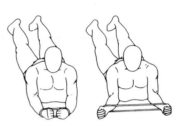

12. PRONE ON ELBOWS EXTERNAL ROTATION

- Lie on your stomach and prop yourself up on your elbows.
- Hold tubing in both hands about shoulder-width apart.
- Pull tubing apart, rotating shoulders outward.
- Hold for 5 seconds.
- Return slowly to starting position.
- Perform ___ sets, ___ repetitions, ___ times/day.

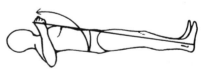

13. EXTERNAL ROTATION AT 90 DEGREES

- Lie down on your back, placing one end of tubing around your foot.
- Raise shoulder 90 degrees up to the side and bend your elbow to 90 degrees.
- Hold tubing in hand and rotate backward as far as you can.
- Return slowly to starting position.
- Perform ___ sets, ___ repetitions, ___ times/day.

Shoulder Acromioclavicular Program

The acromioclavicular (AC) joint is the joint located between the end of your clavicle (collar bone) and the tip of the shoulder (acromion). Injury to this joint can cause tearing of ligaments that stabilize the clavicle and possible separation of the joint. The following strengthening exercises are recommended to stabilize the shoulder joint.

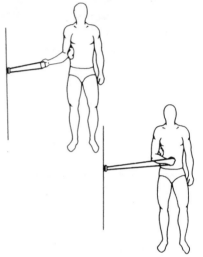

1. INTERNAL ROTATION

- Place tubing in door at elbow level.
- Stand with your involved side toward the door.
- Bend elbow to 90 degrees and place a towel roll between arm and side.
- Hold tubing in hand and rotate shoulder inward toward opposite hip.
- Return slowly to starting position.
- Perform ___ sets, ___ repetitions, ___ times/day.

2. EXTERNAL ROTATION

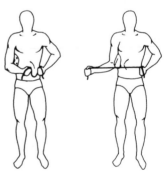

- Wrap tubing around both hands
- Bend elbow of involved arm to 90 degrees and place a towel roll between arm and side.
- Anchor hand of uninvolved shoulder on hip.
- Hold tubing in hand and rotate shoulder outward away from your body.
- Return slowly to starting position.
- Perform ___ sets, ___ repetitions, ___ times/day.

3. EXTENSION IN STANDING

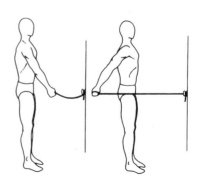

- Place tubing in door at elbow level.
- Face the door, hold tubing in hand of involved side, and pull it straight back behind you, keeping your elbow straight.
- Return slowly to starting position.
- Perform ___ sets, ___ repetitions, ___ times/day.

4. FLEXION

- Stand with one end of tubing under the foot of involved side.
- Hold tubing with thumb on top and lift arm straight up in front of you, keeping elbow straight.
- Return slowly to starting position.
- Perform ___ sets, ___ repetitions, ___ times/day.

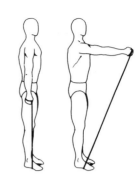

5. ABDUCTION

- Stand with one end of tubing under the foot of involved side.
- Hold tubing with thumb on top and lift arm directly out to the side, keeping elbow straight.
- Return slowly to starting position.
- Perform ___ sets, ___ repetitions, ___ times/day.

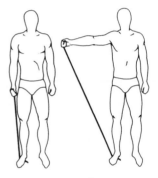

6. HORIZONTAL PULL

- Hold tubing in both hands at shoulder height.
- Pull tubing apart, bringing arms out to each side of your body.
- Return slowly to starting position.
- Perform ___ sets, ___ repetitions, ___ times/day.

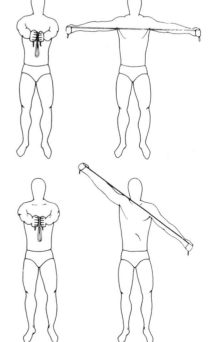

7. DIAGONAL PULL

- Hold tubing in both hands at shoulder height.
- Pull tubing apart at a diagonal, with involved arm moving upward and uninvolved arm moving downward.
- Return slowly to starting position.
- Perform ___ sets, ___ repetitions, ___ times/day.

8 SHOULDER SHRUGS

- Sit or stand with your shoulders back and arms at sides.
- Place weight over top of shoulder or in hand.
- Slowly lift (shrug) shoulder up to ears.
- Hold for 5 seconds. Relax.
- Perform ___ sets, ___ repetitions, ___ times/day.

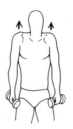
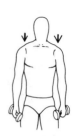

9. EXTENSION IN LYING

- Lie on your stomach, with your involved arm hanging over the side of bed.
- Tie tubing at hand level to object in front of you.
- Hold tubing and pull arm back and up toward ceiling, keeping elbow straight.
- Perform ___ sets, ___ repetitions, ___ times/day.

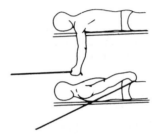
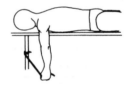

10. HORIZONTAL ABDUCTION

- Lie on your stomach, with your involved arm over the side of bed.
- Tie tubing below shoulder level to stationary object.
- Hold tubing in hand and pull straight out to the side, maintaining shoulder at 90 degrees.
- Return slowly to starting position.
- Perform ___ sets, ___ repetitions, ___ times/day.

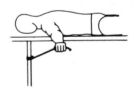

Shoulder Dislocation Program

Shoulder dislocation occurs when the ligaments surrounding your shoulder joint are stretched or torn. This can be caused by direct trauma, such as a fall, or it can be a condition of chronic laxity. To improve stability of the shoulder joint, the following strengthening exercises are recommended.

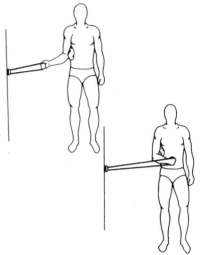

1. INTERNAL ROTATION

- Place tubing in door at elbow level.
- Stand with your involved side toward the door.
- Bend elbow to 90 degrees and place a towel roll between arm and side.
- Hold tubing in hand and rotate shoulder inward toward opposite hip.
- Return slowly to starting position.
- Perform ___ sets, ___ repetitions, ___ times/day.

2. EXTERNAL ROTATION

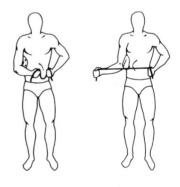

- Wrap tubing around both hands
- Bend elbow of involved arm to 90 degrees and place a towel roll between arm and side.
- Anchor hand of uninvolved shoulder on hip.
- Hold tubing in hand and rotate shoulder outward, away from your body.
- Return slowly to starting position.
- Perform ___ sets, ___ repetitions, ___ times/day.

3. EXTENSION IN STANDING

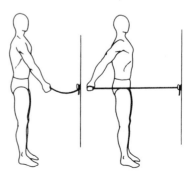

- Place tubing in door at elbow level.
- Face the door, hold tubing in hand of involved side, and pull it straight back behind you, keeping your elbow straight.
- Return slowly to starting position.
- Perform ___ sets, ___ repetitions, ___ times/day.

4. ADDUCTION

- Place tubing in door at hand level.
- Stand with involved arm toward door.
- Hold tubing in hand and pull directly across body, keeping your elbow straight.
- Return slowly to starting position.
- Perform ___ sets, ___ repetitions, ___ times/day.

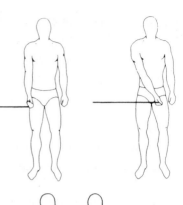

5. FLEXION

- Stand with one end of tubing under the foot of involved side.
- Hold tubing with thumb on top and lift arm straight up in front of you, keeping elbow straight.
- Return slowly to starting position.
- Perform ___ sets, ___ repetitions, ___ times/day.

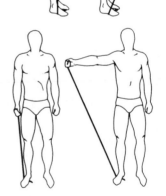

6. ABDUCTION

- Stand with one end of tubing under the foot of involved side.
- Hold tubing with thumb on top and lift arm directly out to the side, keeping elbow straight.
- Return slowly to starting position.
- Perform ___ sets, ___ repetitions, ___ times/day.

7. EMPTY CAN

- Stand with middle of tubing under your feet.
- Hold tubing in both hands, with thumbs turned down.
- Lift your arms up at a thirty degree forward angle, keeping elbows straight.
- Do not lift above shoulder level.
- Return slowly to starting position.
- Perform ___ sets, ___ repetitions, ___ times/day.

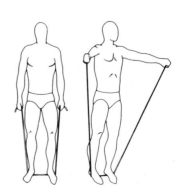

8. HORIZONTAL PULL

- Hold tubing in both hands at shoulder height.
- Pull tubing apart, bringing arms out to each side of your body.
- Return slowly to starting position.
- Perform ___ sets, ___ repetitions, ___ times/day.

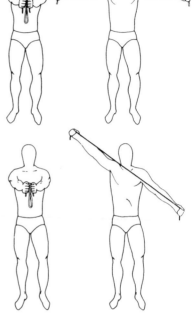

9. DIAGONAL PULL

- Hold tubing in both hands at shoulder height.
- Pull tubing apart at a diagonal, with involved arm moving upward and uninvolved arm moving downward.
- Return slowly to starting position.
- Perform ___ sets, ___ repetitions, ___ times/day.

10. EXTENSION IN LYING

- Lie on your stomach, with your involved arm hanging over the side of bed.
- Tie tubing at hand level to object in front of you.
- Hold tubing and pull arm back and up toward ceiling, keeping elbow straight.
- Return slowly to starting position.
- Perform ___ sets, ___ repetitions, ___ times/day.

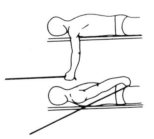

11. HORIZONTAL ABDUCTION

- Lie on your stomach, with your involved arm over the side of bed.
- Tie tubing below shoulder level to stationary object.
- Hold tubing in hand and pull straight out to the side, maintaining shoulder at 90 degrees.
- Return slowly to starting position.
- Perform ___ sets, ___ repetitions, ___ times/day.

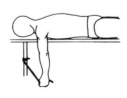

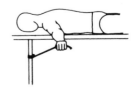

Lateral Epicondylitis Program—Beginning

Tennis elbow is a term commonly used to describe the inflammation on the outer (lateral) side of the elbow due to repeated stress to the area, which results in local elbow pain. The following exercises are recommended to help promote healing and prevent further injury.

1. ISOMETRICS

WRIST EXTENSION

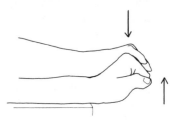

- Place your involved hand over the edge of a table.
- Make a fist, with your palm facing down.
- Move wrist in an upward direction against the resistance of your opposite hand.
- Hold for 5 seconds. Relax.
- Perform ___ sets, ___ repetitions, ___ times/day.

WRIST FLEXION

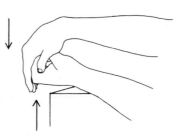

- Place your involved hand over the edge of a table.
- Make a fist, with your palm facing up.
- Move wrist in an upward direction against the resistance of your opposite hand.
- Hold 5 seconds. Relax.
- Perform ___ sets, ___ repetitions, ___ times/day.

RADIAL DEVIATION

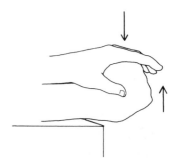

- Place your involved hand over the edge of a table.
- Make a fist, with your thumb facing up.
- Move wrist in an upward direction against the resistance of your opposite hand.
- Hold for 5 seconds. Relax.
- Perform ___ sets, ___ repetitions, ___ times/day.

FINGER EXTENSIONS

- Place your involved hand over the edge of a table.

- Make a fist, with your palm down.

- Move fingers from bent to straightened position against the resistance of your opposite hand.

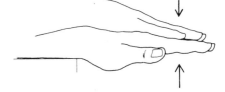

- Hold for 5 seconds. Relax.

- Perform ___ sets, ___ repetitions, ___ times/day.

PRONATION/SUPINATION

- Place your involved hand over the edge of a table.

- Make a fist, with your thumb facing up.

- Rotate your palm downward against the resistance of your opposite hand.

- Repeat by rotating your palm upward.

- Hold for 5 seconds. Relax.

- Perform ___ sets, ___ repetitions, ___ times/day.

2. STRETCHING

WRIST EXTENSION

- With your elbow straight, raise your arm up in front of you to shoulder height, with palm down.

- Bend wrist down and grasp hand with opposite hand.

- Pull back gently until a stretch is felt on the top of the forearm.

- Hold for 20 to 30 seconds. Relax.

- Perform ___ sets, ___ repetitions, ___ times/day.

WRIST FLEXION

- With your elbow straight, raise your arm up in front of you to shoulder height, with palm down.

- Bend wrist up and grasp hand with opposite hand.

- Pull back gently until a stretch is felt on the bottom of the forearm.

- Hold for 20 to 30 seconds. Relax.

- Perform ___ sets, ___ repetitions, ___ times/day.

3. GRIPPING

- Place a tennis ball or racquetball in the palm of your hand.

- Squeeze. Hold for 10 seconds. Relax.

- Perform ___ sets, ___ repetitions, ___ times/day.

Lateral Epicondylitis Program–Advanced

Tennis elbow is a term commonly used to describe the inflammation on the outer (lateral side of the elbow due to repeated stress to the area, which results in local elbow pain. The following exercises are recommended to help promote healing and prevent further injury.

1. WRIST EXTENSION

- Sit in a chair. Place one end of tubing under your foot and hold onto the other end, with palm facing down.

- Support forearm on thigh, with your wrist and hand extended beyond your knee.

- Slowly lift your hand, bending the wrist upward as far as possible.

- Slowly return to starting position.

- Perform ___ sets, ___ repetitions, ___ times/day.

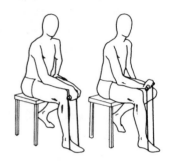

2. WRIST FLEXION

- Sit in a chair.

- Place one end of tubing under your foot and hold onto the other end, with palm facing up.

- Support your forearm on your thigh, with the wrist or hand extended beyond your knee.

- Slowly lift your hand, bending the wrist upward as far as possible.

- Slowly return to starting position.

- Perform ___ sets, ___ repetitions, ___ times/day.

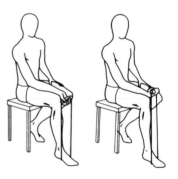

3. FOREARM PRONATION

- Sit in a chair.

- Place one end of tubing under your foot about 10 inches outside the center of your body.

- Hold other end of tubing in your hand, with the palm up.

- Support your forearm on your thigh, with the wrist and hand extended beyond knee.

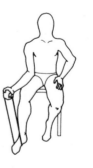
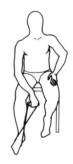

- Slowly rotate your forearm to palm-down position.
- Slowly return to starting position.
- Perform ___ sets, ___ repetitions, ___ times/day.

4. FOREARM SUPINATION

- Sit in a chair.
- Place one end of tubing under your opposite foot and hold the other end in your hand, with the palm down.
- Support your forearm on your thigh, with the wrist and hand extended beyond your knee.
- Slowly rotate your forearm to palm-up position.
- Slowly return to starting position.
- Perform ___ sets, ___ repetitions, ___ times/day.

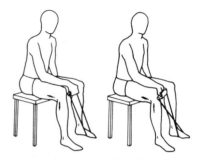

5. RADIAL DEVIATION

- Sit in a chair.
- Place one end of tubing under your foot and hold the other end in your hand, with the thumb facing up.
- Support your forearm on your thigh, with the wrist and hand extended beyond knee.
- Slowly lift your hand, bending the wrist up as far as possible.
- Slowly return to starting position.
- Perform ___ sets, ___ repetitions, ___ times/day.

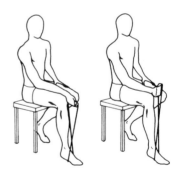

6. ELBOW FLEXION

- Sit in a chair.
- Place one end of tubing under your foot and hold the other end in your hand, with the palm up.
- Support your elbow on your thigh.

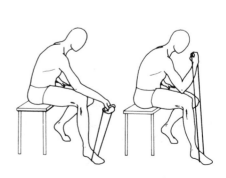

- Slowly bend your elbow up toward you.
- Slowly return to starting position.
- Perform ___ sets, ___ repetitions, ___ times/day.

7. ELBOW EXTENSION

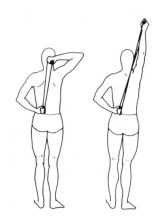

- Stand up.
- Place one end of tubing in your hand and hold the other end with the opposite hand behind your back.
- Straighten the elbow, raising your arm overhead.
- Slowly return to starting position.
- Perform ___ sets, ___ repetitions, ___ times/day.

Patellar Program

Chondromalacia is the diagnosis commonly used to describe a painful condition of the knee caused by traumatic or degenerative changes to the cartilage most commonly located on the undersurface of the patella (kneecap). This condition is associated with a variety of activities that involve repeated bending of the knee, especially if the joint is malaligned. Try to avoid excessive bent knee activities, such as kneeling, stair climbing, and squatting.

1. QUAD SETS

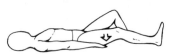

- Lie down on your back.
- Tighten the muscle on the front of your thigh (quadriceps) by pushing the back of your knee into the floor.
- Hold for 5 seconds. Relax.
- Perform ___ sets, ___ repetitions, ___ times/day.

2. STRAIGHT LEG RAISE

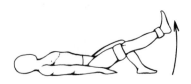

- Lie down on your back.
- Bend up uninvolved knee and place your foot on the floor.
- Tighten the muscle on the front of your thigh on the involved leg (quad set).
- Bring foot of your involved leg toward your face.

- Slowly lift leg 12 to 18 inches off floor, keeping your knee straight.
- Hold for 3 seconds.
- Slowly lower your leg to the floor. Relax.
- Perform ___ sets, ___ repetitions, ___ times/day.

3. HIP ABDUCTION

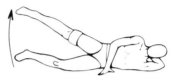

- Lie of your uninvolved side.
- Bend your uninvolved knee slightly for balance.
- Straighten your involved knee and lift your leg 12 to 18 inches toward the ceiling.
- Maintain your hip in the neutral position.
- Hold for 3 seconds.
- Slowly lower leg to the floor. Relax.
- Perform ___ sets, ___ repetitions, ___ times/day.

4. HIP EXTENSION

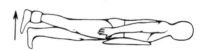

- Lie on your stomach with a pillow under your hips.
- Keeping your knee straight, tighten the muscles on the back of your thigh and buttock.
- Lift your leg toward the ceiling.
- Hold for 3 seconds.
- Slowly lower your leg to the floor. Relax.
- Perform ___ sets, ___ repetitions, ___ times/day.

5. HIP ADDUCTION

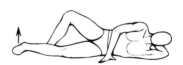

- Lie on your involved side, bending your uninvolved leg.
- Straighten your involved knee, bend your ankle, and raise your leg toward the ceiling.
- Hold for 3 seconds.
- Slowly lower your leg to the floor. Relax.
- Perform ___ sets, ___ repetitions, ___ times/day.

6. HIP FLEXION

- Sit in a straight chair with your knees bent and your feet flat on floor.
- Slowly raise your involved knee toward the ceiling.
- Hold for 3 seconds.
- Slowly lower the knee back to the chair.

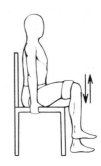

Meniscus Program

The following exercises are recommended for those individuals who may have meniscus (cartilage) damage. The meniscus acts as the main shock absorber of the knee and provides cushioning between the joint surfaces of the femur and the tibia. The meniscus can be strained or town by twisting injuries or chronic overuse from repetitive bending. Avoid repeated knee bending and twisting activities. Let pain be your guide.

1. QUAD SETS

- Lie down on your back.
- Tighten the muscle on the front of your thigh (quadriceps) by pushing the back of your knee into the floor.
- Hold for 5 seconds. Relax.
- Perform ___ sets, ___ repetitions, ___ times/day.

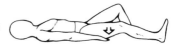

2. STRAIGHT LEG RAISE

- Lie down on your back.
- Bend up your uninvolved knee and place your foot on the floor.
- Tighten the muscle on the front of your thigh on the involved leg (quad set).
- Bring foot of your involved leg toward your face.
- Slowly lift leg 12 to 18 inches off the floor, keeping your knee straight.
- Hold for 3 seconds.
- Slowly lower your leg to the floor. Relax.
- Perform ___ sets, ___ repetitions, ___ times/day.

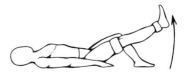

3. HIP ABDUCTION

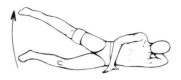

- Lie of your uninvolved side.
- Bend your uninvolved knee slightly for balance.
- Straighten your involved knee and lift the leg 12 to 18 inches toward the ceiling.
- Maintain your hip in the neutral position.
- Hold for 3 seconds.
- Slowly lower your leg to the floor. Relax.
- Perform ___ sets, ___ repetitions, ___ times/day.

4. HIP EXTENSION

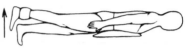

- Lie on your stomach with a pillow under your hips.
- Keeping your knee straight, tighten the muscles on the back of your thigh and buttock. Lift your leg toward the ceiling.
- Hold for 3 seconds.
- Slowly lower your leg to the floor. Relax.
- Perform ___ sets, ___ repetitions, ___ times/day.

5. HAMSTRING CURLS

- Lie on your stomach with a pillow under your hips.
- Slowly bend your involved knee to a 60-degree angle.
- Hold for 3 seconds.
- Slowly lower your leg to the floor. Relax.
- Perform ___ sets, ___ repetitions, ___ times/day.

6. HIP ADDUCTION

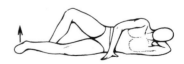

- Lie on your involved side, bending your uninvolved leg and placing it on the floor behind your involved leg..
- Straighten your involved knee and bring the foot toward your face, then raise your leg toward the ceiling.
- Hold for 3 seconds.
- Slowly lower your leg to the floor. Relax.
- Perform ___ sets, ___ repetitions, ___ times/day.

Anterior Cruciate Ligament (ACL) Program

The following exercises are designed for those individuals who have anterior cruciate ligament laxity in the knee. This problem is often caused by acute twist and falling injury, particularly in jumping and twisting activities. Both quadriceps and hamstring strengthening exercises are important in rehabilitation. However, with this particular injury, hamstring strengthening is especially important to stabilize the knee joint.

1. QUAD SETS

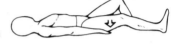

- Lie down on your back.
- Tighten the muscle on the front of your thigh (quadriceps) by pushing the back of your knee into the floor.
- Hold for 5 seconds. Relax.
- Perform ___ sets, ___ repetitions, ___ times/day.

2. STRAIGHT LEG RAISE

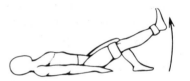

- Lie down on your back.
- Bend up your uninvolved knee and place your foot on the floor.
- Tighten the muscle on the front of your thigh on the involved leg (quad set).
- Bring the foot of your involved leg toward your face.
- Slowly lift your leg 12 to 18 inches off the floor, keeping the knee straight.
- Hold for 3 seconds.
- Slowly lower your leg to the floor. Relax.
- Perform ___ sets, ___ repetitions, ___ times/day.

3. HAMSTRING SETS

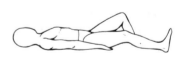

- Lie down on your back, with your involved knee slightly bent over a towel roll.
- Tighten the muscles on the back of your thigh by pulling back with your heel against the floor.
- Hold for 5 seconds. Relax.
- Perform ___ sets, ___ repetitions, ___ times/day.

4. HIP ABDUCTION

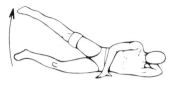

- Lie on your uninvolved side.
- Bend your uninvolved knee slightly for balance.
- Straighten your involved knee and lift your leg 12 to 18 inches toward the ceiling. Maintain your hip in the neutral position.
- Hold for 3 seconds.
- Slowly lower your leg to the floor. Relax.
- Perform ___ sets, ___ repetitions, ___ times/day.

5. HIP EXTENSION

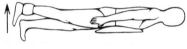

- Lie on your stomach with a pillow under your hips.
- Keeping your knee straight, tighten the muscles on the back of your thigh and buttock.
- Lift your leg toward the ceiling.
- Hold for 3 seconds.
- Slowly lower your leg to the floor. Relax.
- Perform ___ sets, ___ repetitions, ___ times/day.

6. HAMSTRING CURLS

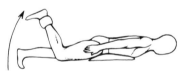

- Lie on your stomach with a pillow under your hips.
- Slowly bend your involved knee to a 60-degree angle.
- Hold for 3 seconds.
- Slowly lower leg to the floor. Relax.
- Perform ___ sets, ___ repetitions, ___ times/day.

7. HIP ADDUCTION

- Lie on your involved side, bending your uninvolved leg and placing it on the floor behind your involved leg..
- Straighten your involved knee and bring the foot toward your face, then raise your leg toward the ceiling.
- Hold for 3 seconds.
- Slowly lower leg to the floor. Relax.
- Perform ___ sets, ___ repetitions, ___ times/day.

Ankle Program

A sprained ankle is a condition of stretched or torn ligaments in your ankle. This is usually caused by a sudden twisting injury. Repetitive ankle sprains can lead to chronic recurrent instability. The following exercises are recommended for rehabilitation and to prevent further injury.

1. ACTIVE RANGE OF MOTION

(A) DORSIFLEXION

- Move ankle upward (toward you) as far as possible.
- Perform ___ sets, ___ repetitions, ___ times/day.

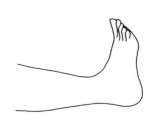

(B) PLANTAR FLEXION

- Move ankle downward (away from you) as far as possible.
- Perform ___ sets, ___ repetitions, ___ times/day.

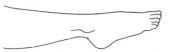

(C) INVERSION

- Move ankle inward as far as possible. Do not rotate hip/knee.
- Perform ___ sets, ___ repetitions, ___ times/day.

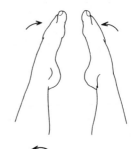

(D) EVERSION

- Move ankle outward as far as possible. Do not rotate hip/knee.
- Perform ___ sets, ___ repetitions, ___ times/day.

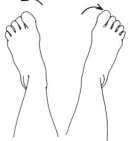

2. CALF STRETCHING

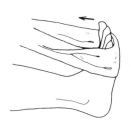

- Hold a towel in both hands, looping the middle of the towel around the ball of your foot.
- Pull towel toward you, moving the foot upward until a stretch is felt in the calf. Keep your knee straight.
- Hold for 20 to 30 seconds. Relax.
- Perform ___ sets, ___ repetitions, ___ times/day.

3. RESISTIVE EXERCISES WITH EXERCISE TUBING

(A) DORSIFLEXION

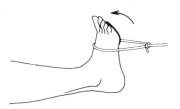

- Tie exercise tubing around a stationary object.
- Place exercise tubing over top of foot. Pull up against it toward face.
- Return slowly to starting position.
- Perform ___ sets, ___ repetitions, ___ times/day.

(B) PLANTAR FLEXION

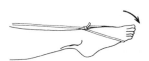

- Hold exercise tubing in both hands, looping the middle of the exercise tubing around the ball of your foot.
- Push foot in a downward direction against the exercise tubing.
- Return slowly to starting position.
- Perform ___ sets, ___ repetitions, ___ times/day.

(C) INVERSION

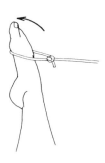

- Tie exercise tubing around a stationary object.
- Place exercise tubing around inside of foot. Pull inward against the tubing. Do not twist hip/knee.
- Return slowly to starting position.
- Perform ___ sets, ___ repetitions, ___ times/day.

(D) EVERSION

- Tie exercise tubing around a stationary object.
- Place exercise tubing around outside of foot. Push outward against the tubing. Do not twist hip/knee.
- Return slowly to starting position.
- Perform ___ sets, ___ repetitions, ___ times/day.

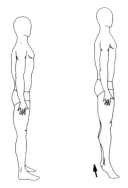

4. TOE RAISES

- Stand with both feet flat on the floor.
- Raise up on both toes. Slowly lower to starting position.
- Progress to one foot on flat surface.
- Progress to both feet off edge of step, then one foot off edge of step.
- Perform ___ sets, ___ repetitions, ___ times/day.

5. GASTROCNEMIUS AND SOLEUS STRETCH

- Face a wall and stand about 2 feet away. Place palms flat against the wall and step forward with one foot, placing the leg to be stretched straight behind you.
- Bend opposite leg and place foot flat on the floor in front of you.
- Keep heel of back leg down and slowly move your hips forward toward the wall, keeping your back straight until a stretch is felt in the calf.
- Hold for 20 to 30 seconds. Relax.
- Repeat the exercise with back leg slightly bent at the knee.
- Perform ___ sets, ___ repetitions, ___ times/day.

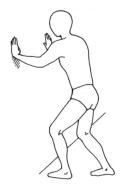

6. BALANCE EXERCISE

- Stand on one leg with your eyes open.
- When able to do this without difficulty for 1 minute, progress to standing on one leg with eyes closed for 1 minute.
- Perform ___ sets, ___ repetitions, ___ times/day.

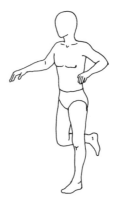

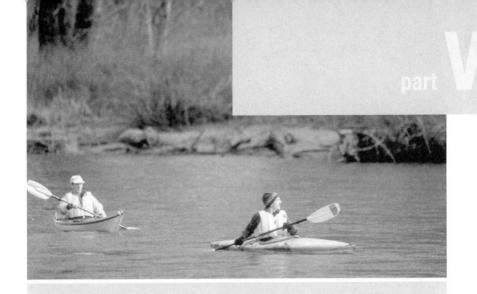

prevention of outdoor recreational injuries

Parts III and IV reviewed specific injuries and rehabilitation. Let's now look at specific ways to avoid reinjury and, more important, prevent the original injury. We'll focus on three different aspects: proper nutrition, use of walking poles, and guidelines for climbing and hiking.

The first chapter is by Laurie Meyer, a dietitian and nutrition consultant. Her nonfad approach to nutrition provides easy-to-follow advice for the recovering fitness enthusiast interested in preventing reinjury, regaining excellent general health, and optimizing weight control.

Tom Rutlin, an expert on walking poles, authors the second chapter. Walking poles reduce stress on the legs by 30 percent and thus represent the perfect bridge between rehabilitation and prevention of injuries.

The third chapter is by John Loliet, coordinator of Pinnacle Peak Park and Trails in Scottsdale, Arizona, who offers practical and helpful advice on how to prevent injuries while climbing and hiking. His essay leads us to the last section of this book, Part VI, which reviews specific orthopedic surgical considerations for joint injuries.

Healthy Eating for Outdoor Recreation

by Laurie Meyer, MS, RD, CD

Good nutrition is essential to living well and being active. Besides tasting good, food provides the fuel your body needs to work and to be active in outdoor recreation. What you eat has a big impact on your overall health and can enhance your ability to enjoy outdoor recreation without increasing the risk of injury or disease.

Eating a healthy diet:

- Maintains normal body functions
- Attains ideal body composition
- Reduces risk factors for disease
- Provides energy to be active
- Minimizes fatigue and injuries

While a good diet keeps the body functioning normally and reduces the risk of many diseases, nutrition for outdoor recreation takes the principles of healthy eating one step further to optimize performance. The quality and the quantity of the foods you eat can have a direct effect on your ability to cope with the physical and mental stress of exercise, whether it's for competition or fun. To prevent injuries, you need a healthy body and a healthy immune system. Eating the right food can fuel your body properly to provide greater endurance, speed, strength, and stamina and encourage better recovery, while keeping the body and immune system healthy.

Before looking at what you should eat, it is important to understand the basic principles of healthy eating.

Eat Breakfast

Breakfast is one of the most important meals. After a 12-hour fast, your body needs fuel. If you eat breakfast, you have a lower chance of obesity, diabetes, and heart disease, and you have better concentration skills and motor abilities. Eating breakfast increases your chance of meeting nutritional requirements for fiber, vitamins, minerals, and phytochemicals.

Eat Regular Meals

Many people skip meals and wait until they have little energy before they refuel. The body needs a supply of energy throughout the day to run properly. Eating regular meals gives you consistent energy and prevents you from getting overly hungry. If you get too hungry, you tend to care less about nutrition and the quality of food and more about satisfying your cravings, so your nutritional status may suffer.

Eat at Regular Times

One of the best ways to keep energy levels high is to eat a meal or snack every 3 to 5 hours. This keeps blood sugar and hormone levels balanced. Skipping meals also puts stress on the body and impairs immune function. Research has shown that people who do not skip meals tend to burn 5 to 10 percent more energy throughout the day, especially when they eat breakfast and lunch.

Eat the Right Amount of Calories

If you do not eat enough calories, you will not have enough energy to work or to play. Skimping on calories can also sabotage your weight because you will burn muscle instead of fat. Include the right mix of carbohydrates, proteins, and fats at meals and snacks to produce optimal energy for your body type and activity level, whether you are running, hiking, skiing, or climbing.

Aim for Variety

Don't eat the same foods every day or at every meal. Eat a variety of foods, including fruits, vegetables, whole grains, legumes, meats, poultry, fish, dairy foods, and healthy fats, to give you all of the nutrients your body needs to stay healthy and active, regardless of which outdoor activity you pursue.

Eat Wholesome Foods

Choose natural, whole foods over processed foods whenever you can because they not only provide more vitamins, minerals, antioxidants, and fiber, but also make you feel more satisfied afterwards. Minimize junk foods like candy, chips, and fast foods because they are low in nutrients and may contain compounds that are hazardous to your health.

Drink Fluids

Every organ and system in the body requires water to function. Muscle building, muscle breakdown, and muscle contraction are all affected by fluid balance. Dehydration impairs health and performance. Drink water or other fluids throughout the day before you get thirsty to maintain hydration. This is vital for long-distance activities like running, biking, climbing, and hiking.

Metabolic Differences

Healthy eating is not necessarily a one-for-all prescription. It depends on a lot of different things, including your genetic makeup, lifestyle, goals, and personal requirements.

There no longer is one standard diet that is recommended for everyone because it is now understood that we all have metabolic and biochemical differences based on our genetics. Since we are different in ways our bodies process foods and utilize nutrients, we may require different diets to achieve optimal health and performance. We all need the same types of nutrients, but some people may need higher amounts of protein or fat to stay healthy, while others need more carbohydrates. Listen to your body and see what works best for you.

Nutritional Goals

Your chief nutritional goal should be these:

- Eat adequate calories
- Eat appropriate foods to obtain the right mix of nutrients
- Drink fluids to stay hydrated
- Eat at the right times to enhance performance

Caloric Requirements

All food is made up of carbohydrates, protein, and fat, which supply the body with energy in the form of calories. The body uses various enzymes and water to convert the food we eat into usable sugars, amino acids, and fatty acids. Getting the right number of calories for your body and activity level promotes peak performance while maintaining good health. The more muscle mass you have, the more fuel you need. If you don't get enough calories, you may lose muscle mass and increase the risk of or injury. Eating too few calories increases the risk of infection.

CALCULATING CALORIES

There are several methods used to calculate caloric requirements. Some are very complex, but all give similar results. Here is an easy and accurate way to determine your basal energy requirements, or the number of calories your body needs at rest.

Body weight* (in pounds) x 10–12 (calorie factor) = basal energy requirements

Example:

125-pound female

125 $\times$ 10 = 1,250 calories   125 $\times$ 12 = 1,500 calories

basal energy requirement = 1,250 to 1,500 calories a day

*If you are overweight, use your estimated healthy target weight in pounds.

All activity increases your caloric requirements. Energy is needed to supply your working muscles with fuel. To determine how many calories you need for work, exercise, or outdoor recreation, multiply your basal energy requirements by an activity factor from the chart below.

Activity	Activity Factor	Example
Very light activity	1.3–1.4	Slow hiking
Light activity	1.4–1.6	Biking
Moderate activity	1.6–1.8	Cross-country skiing
Heavy activity	1.8–2.0	Long-distance running, mountain climbing

Basal energy requirement x (activity factor) = daily calorie requirement

Example:

125-pound moderately active female

1,500 calories $\times$ 1.6 = 2,400 calories a day

Active people consuming less than 2,000 calories a day may have a difficult time meeting nutritional needs, particularly for iron and calcium. Weight loss, glycogen depletion, and dehydration are all possible results of an inadequate diet.

Carbohydrates

The main benefits of carbohydrates:

- Digest quickly
- Supply immediate energy
- Replenish glycogen stores

Carbohydrates are the chief source of energy. The body prefers to use carbohydrates as fuel for most activities. If you don't consume enough carbohydrates, your muscles will tire quickly, and you won't have the energy to last during a prolonged activity like rock climbing, mountain biking, or paddling.

Carbohydrates are digested and broken down in the body into glucose for immediate energy. When we start exercising, our main fuel source is glucose. However, only a very small amount of glucose is available in the bloodstream, so the body relies on a type of stored energy called glycogen.

Glycogen, which is essential for optimum performance, has these qualities:

- Long chains of glucose
- Stored in liver and muscle
- Provides energy to working muscles
- Needed during high-intensity exercise

Glycogen is made from carbohydrates and converted to long chains of sugar molecules. It is stored in the liver and muscle in limited amounts for later use. When you run low on blood sugar during an endurance effort, your body dips into liver glycogen reserves and supplies the blood and ultimately the brain with fuel. Your muscles then use up their own supply of stored glycogen. You have enough stored glycogen in your muscles to last for about 90 minutes of vigorous exercise, like running and biking.

If exercise continues, your body drains glycogen from your muscles. After 30 minutes of activity, the heart pumps faster and the body begins to use fatty acids stored in adipose tissue, along with glucose from glycogen stores and a very small amount of protein in the form of amino acids.

Exercising muscles take sugar out of the bloodstream, causing blood sugar levels to drop. This sets off a chain reaction that makes you experience extreme fatigue. Glycogen stores must be replaced during any activity that lasts longer than 90 minutes, or you will run out of fuel and "hit the wall." Consuming some form of carbohydrate 30 minutes into your workout will help you to exercise longer and more intensely if your activity lasts more than 90 minutes.

Regular carbohydrate consumption also keeps immunity high. Some studies have shown immunity drops with long, intense exercise, such as marathon running and century bike riding, unless you consume carbohydrates during exercise.

TYPES OF CARBOHYDRATES

Carbohydrates come from plant sources and are converted into energy by the body. Even though the body converts all forms of carbohydrates into glucose, they aren't equal when it comes to the nutrients and the energy they provide.

Simple carbohydrates are made up of single sugar molecules. They tend to be digested and absorbed more quickly into the bloodstream for quick energy, but this is only temporary. Because your body absorbs simple sugars quickly, they also leave your system fast.

Examples of Simple Carbohydrates:

- Sugar
- Honey
- Maple syrup
- Fruit
- Fruit juice
- Candy
- Soft drinks

Many simple sugars are referred to as "empty calories" because they provide calories but few nutrients. New evidence indicates that eating a diet that is high in simple sugars can lead to health problems, including periodontal disease, hypoglycemia, diabetes, a weakened immune system, colon cancer, heart disease, and vision problems.

Complex carbohydrates, also called starches, are made of sugar molecules that are linked together. They are usually digested and absorbed into the bloodstream more slowly to provide a steady supply of energy. Foods high in complex carbohydrates often contain more B vitamins, potassium, magnesium, iron, and calcium. These nutrients are needed for energy production and muscle contraction and are often depleted during physical activity. Whole grains, legumes, and vegetables supply greater amounts of B vitamins, potassium, and magnesium than refined starches.

Examples of Complex Carbohydrates:

- Breads
- Cereals
- Grains
- Pasta
- Vegetables
- Legumes
- Milk

There is new evidence that not all simple sugars provide quick energy, and not all complex carbohydrates provide sustained energy. Some simple carbohydrates, like table sugar, enter the bloodstream quickly, while honey and fruit enter the bloodstream more slowly. Some complex carbohydrates enter the bloodstream faster than simple carbohydrates. White bread and snack crackers, both complex carbohydrates, are absorbed very quickly. Many of these refined carbohydrates are suspected of increasing the risk of obesity and diabetes. Oatmeal and kidney beans are complex carbohydrates that provide a steady source of energy and are rich in vitamins and minerals.

GLYCEMIC INDEX

While this may sound confusing, it's not. A new and better way to classify carbohydrates, called the glycemic index, can help you determine which carbohydrates are best for you when you are active and when you are not.

The glycemic index (GI) ranks foods according to how they affect blood sugar levels. The GI measures the rate carbohydrates are digested and absorbed and the amount of insulin released in the bloodstream. It tells you whether a food will raise blood sugar levels dramatically, moderately, or just a little. High blood sugar and insulin levels are responsible for many diseases, including obesity, diabetes, high blood pressure, heart disease, stroke, and certain cancers. There are three categories:

High GI Foods:

- Digest quickly
- Spike blood glucose and insulin levels
- Stimulate appetite
- Increase fat storage
- Raise blood pressure, heart disease, type 2 diabetes

Medium GI Foods:

- Digest moderately
- Maintain blood glucose levels
- Maintain appetite

Low GI Foods:

- Digest slowly
- Gradual rise in blood glucose
- Improve sensitivity to insulin
- Curb appetite
- Aid weight loss
- Stabilize diabetes
- Lower blood lipids

Table 2 rates common foods using the glycemic index.

TABLE 2. GLYCEMIC INDEX

High GI (70 or more)		Medium GI (between 55 and 69)		Low GI (54 or less)	
Dates	103	Whole wheat bread	69	Sweet potato	54
French bread	95	Taco shell	68	Sourdough bread	54
Baked potato	93	Grape nuts cereal	67	Pumpernickel bread	49
Cornflakes	84	Pineapple	66	Oatmeal	49
Pretzels	83	Cantaloupe	65	Chocolate bar	49
Rice cake	82	Couscous	65	Orange	43
Jelly beans	80	Table sugar	64	Spaghetti	41
Vanilla wafers	77	Rye bread	64	Apple	36
Waffle	76	Raisins	64	Yogurt, fruit	33
Total	76	Beets	64	Skim milk	32
French fries	75	Bran muffin	60	Kidney beans	27
Doughnut	75	Honey	60	Grapefruit	25
Graham crackers	74	Basmati rice	58	Barley	25
Corn chips	72	Oatmeal cookie	57	Whole milk	22
Watermelon	72	Pita bread	56	Soybeans	18
Bagel	72	Popcorn	55	Peanuts	10
White bread	70	Banana	55	Broccoli	10

GI = glycemic index

Many people benefit from high GI foods both during and after strenuous activity. Before an activity, it is best to eat low GI foods, such as pasta and oatmeal, because they are digested and absorbed more slowly and supply glucose to working muscles without causing nausea or fatigue during exercise. But both during and after exercise or outdoor recreational activities, high GI foods are preferred because they replace more glycogen in your muscles.

Foods with a low GI are often recommended to prevent disease. You don't have to eliminate all high GI foods, but rather balance your diet by including more low and medium GI foods at meals and snacks.

CARBOHYDRATE REQUIREMENTS

Carbohydrate requirements range from 40 to 70 percent of calories, depending on metabolic type and level of activity. For optimal outdoor recreational activities, aim for 55 to 60 percent carbohydrate calories. Eating less than this could risk depletion of glycogen stores, which will severely affect your performance.

Eating enough carbohydrates also allows you to perform back-to-back days of exercise, whether it is climbing, hiking, or skiing. If you feel exhausted the day after participating in an activity, it may be a sign you aren't eating enough carbohydrates.

Example:

1,500 calories × 60% = 900 carbohydrate calories ÷ 4 calories/gram
= 225 grams of carbohydrate

One serving of a carbohydrate-rich food provides about 15 grams of carbohydrate.

One carbohydrate serving equals:

- 1 slice of bread
- 1 piece of fruit
- ½ cup cooked cereal or grain
- ¾ cup cold cereal
- 1 medium potato
- 1 glass of milk, or yogurt
- 2 cups of green vegetables

The timing of your meal is as important as eating enough carbohydrates for optimal performance during outdoor recreational activities.

Before Activity:

- Eat a carbohydrate-rich diet the week before to ensure adequate glycogen stores.
- Good Sources:
    - Spaghetti marinara
    - Oatmeal and milk
    - Bean burrito

During Activity:

- Activities lasting less than 90 minutes do not require refueling during the activity.
- Activities lasting longer than 90 minutes require 30 to 60 grams of carbohydrates every hour to maintain blood glucose levels.

- Good Sources:
    - High-GI carbohydrate sports bars
    - Sports drinks
    - Banana
    - Raisins

After Activity:

- Eat high-GI carbohydrates within 2 hours for faster recovery.
- Combine protein with carbohydrate to increase carbohydrate absorption.
- Good Sources:
    - Turkey and tomato sandwich on a bagel
    - French bread pizza
    - Baked potato stuffed with chicken, broccoli, and cheese

Protein

The chief features of protein:

- Made of amino acids
- Builds and repairs muscle
- Essential for all body functions

Protein is not a primary fuel source but is needed to build, maintain, and repair muscles and organs. Protein is made of amino acids and is needed to manufacture hemoglobin, which takes oxygen to all cells; antibodies, which fight off infection and disease; and enzymes and hormones, which regulate body functions. The body cannot store protein, so you need to consume it every day. When you do eat protein, it goes to where it is needed the most.

Eating more than the recommended amount of protein does not improve body functions, or make stronger, larger muscles. Extra protein burdens the kidneys and liver and is stored as fat, not as muscle. Too much protein impairs performance and increases injuries. High-protein diets deplete glycogen stores more quickly, making you feel tired and sluggish.

Eating too little protein will also affect your health and performance. If you train hard, you need more protein. If you follow a low-calorie diet, you also need higher protein levels. Protein is especially important after a workout or activity when your body repairs muscle damage and shuttles energy back to your muscles.

PROTEIN REQUIREMENTS

Normal requirement:	0.37 gram protein/pound body weight
Endurance and long-distance activities:	0.55 gram protein/pound body weight
Body-building activities:	0.82 gram protein/pound body weight

Example:

125-pound active female

0.55 × 125 pounds = 69 grams of protein

Seven to eight grams of protein can be found in:

- 1 egg
- 1 oz. meat
- 1 oz. poultry
- 1 oz. fish
- 1 oz. cheese
- 1 cup milk or yogurt
- ½ cup legumes
- 2 tbsp. peanut butter

If you eat sufficient calories, protein intake is usually adequate, and protein supplementation is not necessary, provided you eat a variety of foods and include good protein sources in your diet.

Protein is made from twenty different amino acids. The body can manufacture ten amino acids but the other ten are considered essential and must be included in our diet every day.

High-Quality Protein Sources:

- Eggs
- Red meat
- Poultry
- Fish
- Seafood
- Milk
- Cheese
- Soybeans

Include animal and soy foods in your diet every day to obtain high-quality protein. Fermented soy foods such as tempeh, natto, and miso are the best tolerated.

Low-Quality Protein Sources:

- Grains
- Legumes
- Vegetables
- Nuts
- Seeds

Grains, beans, vegetables, nuts, and seeds are considered lower quality proteins because they are missing one or more of the essential amino acids, but they do provide enough additional protein to meet daily requirements.

EGGS ARE OK

Eggs are the highest quality protein and contain iron, zinc, choline, and lutein. They support a healthy immune system and protect the brain and memory. Eggs do not raise cholesterol levels in most people. Type 1 diabetics do not metabolize cholesterol well, so they should limit egg consumption. The rest of us can safely eat eggs every day.

RED MEAT HAS IMPORTANT NUTRIENTS

Red meats supply many important nutrients that are difficult to obtain from other foods. Beef, pork, lamb, and turkey legs are good sources of iron, zinc, and B vitamins. These nutrients are needed for a healthy immune system, energy production, exercise performance, wound healing, and a healthy nervous system. These nutrients are especially needed during heavy training or exhausting activities. Include several servings of red meat or turkey legs each week. Choose lean cuts of meat, such as tenderloin, sirloin, round, and chuck.

You may also try grass-fed beef, bison, and venison because they are lower in overall fat and contain special fats called omega-3 fatty acids that reduce inflammation and conjugated linolenic acids that lower cancer risk and obesity.

INCLUDE DAIRY FOODS

Dairy foods supply calcium, needed for bone health, weight control, normal heart rhythm, and blood pressure. Aim for three servings of dairy foods daily, including milk, yogurt, and cheese. While calcium is necessary to reduce bone fractures, it must be balanced with magnesium for the best utilization. Magnesium is found in whole grains, leafy vegetables, and legumes.

Fat

The main benefits of fat:

- Concentrated energy source
- Absorbs and transports nutrients
- Supports brain function
- Protects organs
- Maintains immune system
- Boosts endurance

Fat is not bad for you. It adds flavor to food and helps you to feel satisfied. Many fats, such as those found in chocolate, nuts, and olive oil, have health benefits. Fat supplies 2¼ times more energy than either protein or carbohydrates. It helps the body absorb and use fat-soluble vitamins and supplies essential fatty acids required to maintain normal body function, especially in the brain. Eating too little healthy fat affects mood and increases anger and depression.

The body stores fat beneath the skin, around the organs, and inside the muscles. While blood glucose and muscle glycogen provide working muscles with most of their energy, the body uses fat when exercising for longer periods of time, lasting over 30 minutes. Research has found the right amount and type of fat in the diet can boost endurance and immunity and keep your joints well lubricated.

Fat does not cause weight gain. Eating too many calories increases weight. Some people eat large portions of fat-free foods because they think they are healthier. Nothing could be further from the truth. Fat-free foods tend to be high in sugar and refined carbohydrates and often are higher in calories.

FAT REQUIREMENTS

Eating the right fats at the right time can make a difference in how you perform and how you feel. Fat should supply no less than 20 percent of calories and preferably at least 30 percent of total calories, especially if you are very active. Endurance training turns muscles into better fat burners, which increases the requirement for fat. Runners, hikers, and other athletes with higher calorie needs should get at least 30 percent fat calories to meet their energy requirements.

Example:

1,500 calorie requirement × 30% fat = 450 fat calories ÷ 9 calories/gram = 50 grams of fat

Four to five grams of fat can be found in:

- 1 tsp. butter or oil
- 2 tsp. salad dressing
- 2 oz. fish
- 1 oz. meat
- ½ oz. cheese
- 5–6 nuts

Low-fat diets may lower immune function along with endurance and are often lacking in essential nutrients like protein, iron, and zinc.

Fat slows down the amount of oxygen to your muscles for up to 2 hours after you ingest it. When you exercise, you want to make sure you give your muscles as much oxygen as possible, so avoid eating high-fat meals or snacks before an event or outdoor recreational activity. More fat can be consumed afterwards and on nonexercise days.

TYPES OF FAT

There are four types of fat:

- Polyunsaturated fatty acids
- Monounsaturated fatty acids
- Saturated fatty acids
- Trans fatty acids

The molecular arrangement of fatty acids will determine whether a fat is classified as polyunsaturated, monounsaturated, saturated, or trans.

Polyunsaturated Fatty Acids

The chief features of polyunsaturated fats:

- Regulate metabolism
- Maintain healthy immune system
- Regulate cell growth
- Maintain brain function

Omega-6 fatty acids and omega-3 fatty acids are polyunsaturated fats considered essential because the body cannot make them. Essential fats make hormone-like substances that regulate cellular metabolism, build a strong immune system, regulate growth, maintain heart health, promote healthy skin and nerve fibers, and prevent tumor growth.

Omega-6 Sources:

- Corn oil
- Safflower oil
- Soybean oil
- Sunflower oil
- Sesame oil
- Nuts
- Seeds

While omega-6 fatty acids are necessary for good health, eating too many omega-6 fats can upset metabolic balance, resulting in increased inflammation, blood clots, and insulin resistance, and impaired mental function and bone health. Currently, Americans eat too many omega-6 fatty acids and not enough omega-3 fatty acids. This imbalance is responsible for the rise in many degenerative diseases.

Omega-3 fatty acids are crucial to good health. Our early ancestors ate much more omega-3 fat than we do today. Instead, we eat mostly polyunsaturated omega-6 fatty acids and trans fatty acids from processed and fried foods. Many chronic diseases may have developed as a result, including autoimmune disease, heart disease, some cancers, multiple sclerosis, and skin conditions like psoriasis and eczema. Omega-3 fatty acids also have potent anti-inflammatory properties, making them especially important for anyone who is active.

Omega-3 Sources:

- Cold water fish
- Cod liver oil
- Flaxseed
- Chia seed
- Walnuts
- Canola oil
- High omega-3 eggs
- Grass-fed meat
- Grass-fed dairy
- Bison
- Venison
- Green leafy vegetables

The ratio of omega-6 to omega-3 fatty acids in early humans was believed to be about 1:1 to 2:1. Currently, most Americans consume an omega-6 to omega-3 fatty acid ratio of 20:1 or greater. For optimum health and fitness, increase your consumption of omega-3 fatty acid foods, and eat fewer omega-6 fatty acid foods.

Monounsaturated Fatty Acids

The chief features of monounsaturated fatty acids:

- Reduce inflammation
- Antioxidant activity
- Lower LDL cholesterol
- Maintain HDL cholesterol

Monounsaturated fats are considered the healthiest because they exhibit natural antioxidant activity, help lower low-density lipoproteins (LDL, or bad cholesterol), and maintain high-density lipoproteins (HDL or good cholesterol), reduce inflammation, and help to reduce heart disease, cancer, and diabetes. The majority of the fat in the diet should come from monounsaturated fats.

Monounsaturated Fat Sources:

- Olives and olive oil
- Macadamia nut oil
- Avocado and avocado oil
- Peanuts and peanut oil
- Most nuts
- Canola oil

Olive oil reduces inflammation and protects against heart disease, cancer, and stomach ulcers. It is a rich source of antioxidants and phytochemicals. Extra virgin olive oil provides the most benefit.

Canola oil is highly refined and deodorized and produces trans fatty acids when heated. When ingested, this increases inflammation in the body, so it may not be a good choice for most people, especially athletes and active people.

Saturated Fatty Acids

The chief features of saturated fatty acids:

- Stable
- Help utilize calcium
- Antimicrobial properties
- Lower Lp(a)
- Balance omega-3 fats

A small amount of saturated fat is necessary in the diet. Saturated fatty acids constitute at least 50 percent of all cell membranes and are needed to effectively incorporate calcium in the skeletal structure. The fatty acids found in butter, coconut, and palm oil have antimicrobial properties that protect the digestive tract against harmful microorganisms.

Saturated fats do not cause heart disease. The majority of the fat found in clogged arteries is polyunsaturated, not saturated. Heart disease should not be blamed on animal fats or cholesterol, but rather on hydrogenated trans fats, oxidized fats, chemically treated fats, vitamin and mineral deficiencies, and refined carbohydrates. Saturated fats actually lower lipoprotein (a), a measure of heart disease risk in the blood, and allow the body to utilize omega-3 fatty acids. Stearic and palmitic acids, both saturated fats, are the preferred fuel for the heart.

Saturated Fat Sources:

- Butter
- Dairy fats
- Meat fats
- Coconut oil
- Palm oil
- Chocolate

Butter contains vitamins A, D, and E. Butter produced from cows eating grasses is the healthiest because it has a balance of omega-3 and omega-6 fatty acids. Butter also contains conjugated linolenic acid, which may reduce cancer and tumor cell growth, diabetes, and obesity, especially abdominal fat.

Coconut oil is a healthy saturated fat as long as it is extra virgin or unrefined. Coconut oil is very stable and can be used in cooking at high temperatures. Unrefined coconut oil does not raise LDL cholesterol or contribute to heart disease, but it does reduce symptoms of digestive disorders, support the immune system, help to prevent bacterial, viral, and fungal infections, and may improve thyroid function.

Chocolate contains stearic acid, which does not raise cholesterol or heart disease risk. Dark chocolate contains flavonoids that may reduce cell damage and boost the immune system

Trans Fatty Acids

The chief features of trans fatty acids:

- Hydrogenated oils
- Raise LDL cholesterol
- Lower HDL cholesterol

- Raise Lp(a)
- Increase heart attack and stroke
- Increase diabetic complications

Fats and oils injected with hydrogen gas at high temperatures under high pressure are made into solids to make them more stable. This is called hydrogenation and converts unsaturated fatty acids to trans fatty acids. Unfortunately, trans fatty acids are responsible for many serious health problems and diseases, including cancer, heart disease, diabetic complications, obesity, immune system dysfunction, birth defects, hormonal imbalance, and bone problems.

Cooking oils heated to high temperatures, such as in sautéing, stir-frying, and deep-frying, produce mutagenic substances and trans fatty acids that weaken the immune system and increase inflammation. The oils most susceptible are polyunsaturated fats.

Trans Fatty Acid Sources:

- Hydrogenated fats and oils
- Margarine
- Shortening
- Deep-fried foods
- Commercial bakery
- Snack chips and crackers
- Processed cheese

Use healthful fats in place of trans fats. Snack on nuts instead of potato chips. Use avocado instead of margarine spread on bread and sandwiches. Cook with olive oil instead of shortening. Add flaxseeds to salads, cooked cereals, and smoothies.

Water

The benefits of water:

- Carries nutrients to cells
- Removes waste
- Cools body
- Maintains muscle function

HYDRATION

Up to 70 percent of the human body is water. It is essential for good health, especially if you are active. Water brings valuable oxygen and nutrients into the cells and carries away carbon dioxide and other waste products. Every organ and body system requires water. Muscle building, breakdown, and contraction are all affected by fluid status. Water also lubricates joints. Water that is used during metabolism or eliminated in urine and sweat must be replaced regularly.

One of the most important functions of water is to cool the body. When the body gets hot, it sweats, and as the sweat evaporates, the body is cooled. If fluids are not replaced, the fluid balance is disrupted, and the body may overheat. Humid days require more fluids. If the air is humid, sweat does not evaporate, and the body is not cooled. This can lead to overheating and heat disorders that may require medical attention.

LACK OF FLUIDS

Early fatigue, headache, and dizziness are signs of dehydration. Thirst is not always a good indicator of fluid needs if you are active. You need to drink before, during, and after any sport or outdoor recreational activity. If you are exhausted afterwards, chances are you didn't drink enough.

FLUID REQUIREMENTS

It is estimated we lose 8 to 12 cups of water each day. Drinking less than that amount can damage the body. Most people need a minimum of 2 quarts of water or other fluids every day. More is needed in hot, humid weather and during exercise. If you are overweight, drink 1 additional cup for every 25 pounds of excess weight.

Before Activity:

- Drink 12 to 16 oz. 1 to 2 hours before activity.
- Drink 4 to 6 oz. 10 to 15 minutes before activity.

During Activity:

- Drink 4 to 6 oz. every 15 to 20 minutes.

After Activity:

- Drink 16 oz. for every pound of weight loss.

REPLACE FLUIDS

Drinking water is the easiest way to replace body fluids. Plain cold water is the best and most economical source of fluid. The body absorbs cold fluids faster than warmer ones. Sport drinks are recommended for activities lasting longer than 60 minutes or during any intense activity. These drinks should be between 6 and 8 percent carbohydrate or 15 to 18 grams of carbohydrate per cup.

You can also replace body fluids with foods containing a lot of water, such as oranges, peaches, watermelon, apples, grapes, lettuce, and tomatoes. These foods provide water and carbohydrates that replace both fluids and energy lost during activity.

Preventing Injuries

If you are feeling sluggish or fatigued you may be training too hard, be dehydrated, not be eating enough calories or eating too few carbohydrates. You can minimize muscle cramps and muscle soreness by changing your diet.

Muscle cramps plague many fitness enthusiasts, especially during warm weather. These painful spasms usually strike either during a long session of exercise or soon after you finish. The cause of exercise-induced cramping may be due to dehydration from heavy sweating on hot days and loss of electrolytes.

Muscle fatigue may be the real culprit behind cramping. Fatigue brings on a series of internal changes that cause your muscle to enter a state of enhanced excitability, shortening the muscle and causing pain. The muscle relaxes after 5 to 15 seconds, but passive stretching of the cramped muscle can bring immediate relief, since the stretch interrupts the excitability cycle and helps your muscle get rest.

To prevent muscle cramps:

- Eat adequate carbohydrates
- Drink enough fluids
- Stretch

Make sure you drink fluids and consume carbohydrates during workouts lasting 60 minutes or longer. Eating a banana, a handful of dried fruit, or an energy bar and drinking plenty of water during a workout will help delay muscle fatigue.

MUSCLE SORENESS

Exercise causes small tears in muscles, which allow the muscle to grow. To repair these small tears, your immune system responds with inflammation. The swelling puts pressure on nearby nerves, causing pain. It is common to have mild discomfort after a tough exercise session. Damaged muscle cells bring on inflammation and soreness, which makes your next workout feel harder than it should.

To reduce muscle soreness:

- Increase antioxidants
- Increase omega-3 fats

Antioxidants

Antioxidants are found abundantly in fruits and vegetables and whole grains. They prevent free radical damage in your muscles. Free radicals are out-of-control molecules that cause cell and tissue damage and are one of the causes of postexercise pain. Free radicals are all around us. Cigarette smoke, volatile chemicals, household chemicals, pesticides, ultraviolet rays, heated cooking oils, and injuries all produce free radicals. Burning glucose and fat for energy during exercise also produces free radicals. Active people need more antioxidant-rich foods to reduce inflammation, soreness, and muscle damage.

- Eat eight to ten servings of fruits and vegetables a day—the more colorful and varied, the better.
- Eat six or more servings of whole grains, such as barley, millet, quinoa, and buckwheat.
- Vitamin E is a powerful antioxidant that may help protect you from the oxidative damage caused by endurance exercise. It is found in nuts, seeds, and oils. During heavy periods of training, a vitamin E supplement containing 400 IU of mixed tocopherols may be beneficial. Take it with a meal to enhance absorption.

Scientists at the U.S. Department of Agriculture Human Research Center on Aging measured the sum antioxidant power from vitamins C and E, carotenes, selenium, and phytochemicals found in fruits and vegetables. The following foods have the greatest antioxidant activity. Try to include more of these foods in your diet.

Highest Antioxidant Foods:

- Kale
- Prunes
- Spinach
- Oranges
- Concord grape juice
- Blueberries
- Strawberries
- Kiwi
- Mushrooms
- Tomato juice

- Raisins
- Sweet potato
- Orange juice
- Red bell pepper
- Brussels sprouts
- Red grapefruit
- Tomato

Omega-3 Fats

Omega-3 fats have natural anti-inflammatory activity, which helps to reduce muscle pain. Fish oil is the best source of omega-3 fatty acids. Rather than take supplements, you can eat oily fish at least three or four times a week.

Best Omega-3 Fatty Acid Sources:

- Salmon
- Sardines
- Halibut
- Whitefish
- Trout
- Light tuna
- Tilapia
- Cod liver oil

Summary

Eating a balanced diet is necessary to maintain good health and to reduce the risk of chronic disease.

A healthy diet also gives you the extra energy and nutrients needed to enjoy leisure time and outdoor recreational activities without the risk of injury or illness. Eating adequate calories to fuel your body is necessary, along with getting the right mix of nutrients. This can be accomplished by eating a variety of healthful foods. Carbohydrates are critical to fuel working muscles engaged in outdoor recreational activities. Eating too little carbohydrate not only will result in early fatigue, but can also increase the risk of injury and infection. Likewise, while daily protein intake is necessary for building and repairing muscles, eating an extremely high-protein diet can impair performance and increase injury by depleting glycogen stores. Drinking enough fluids is extremely important. Every organ and body system depends on water to function normally, and this becomes even more important when engaging in outdoor recreational activities to avoid dehydration.

Eating healthfully is not that difficult to do. It can be accomplished by following these commonsense principles.

- Eat a variety of wholesome, natural foods throughout the day.
- Eat more fruits and vegetables to obtain important nutrients.
- Eat more whole grains and fewer processed and convenience foods.
- Eat a high-quality protein source every day.
- Include healthy fats in your daily diet.
- Drink plenty of fluids to maintain hydration.

By following these simple guidelines, you will have the energy and health to live your life to its fullest potential and enjoy all of your favorite outdoor recreational activities.

Bibliography

Applegate, L. *Encyclopedia of Sports and Fitness Nutrition.* Roseville, California: Prima Publishing, 2002.

Brand-Miller, J., T. Wolever, S. Colagiuri, and K. Foster-Powell. *The Glucose Revolution: The Authoritative Guide to the Glycemic Index—The Groundbreaking Medical Discovery.* New York: Marlowe & Co., 1999.

Erasmus, U. *Fats That Heal, Fats That Kill.* Burnaby, British Columbia: Alive Books, 1993.

Rosenbloom, C. A. *Sports Nutrition: A Guide for the Professional Working with Active People.* Chicago: Sports and Cardiovascular Nutrition Group and The American Dietetic Association, 2000.

Wolcott W., and T. Fahey. *The Metabolic Typing Diet.* New York: Broadway Books, 2002.

Laurie Meyer is a registered dietitian and body ecologist with a nutrition consulting practice in Milwaukee, Wisconsin, where she works with individuals, industry, and the media. Meyer is a former national spokesperson for the American Dietetic Association and has contributed to hundreds of articles and books on nutrition and fitness. She appears weekly on the Milwaukee NBC news, providing insight on the latest nutrition research, and is currently working on a quick and healthy cookbook.

Use of Poles for Fitness Walking, Hiking/Trekking, Sports Training, and Rehabilitation

by Tom Rutlin

The Evolution of "Fitness Poles"

On a long journey, a walking stick can help propel the body, add balance, take some of the stress off joints, and provide relief to tired muscles. Over thousands of years walkers have simply selected a strong tree branch and fashioned a walking stick according to their own taste and requirements.

The evolution of modern walking poles, which are used in pairs, can be traced to the very early days of skiing. Early skis were very long, often as much as 12 feet long. They were not designed for recreation; rather, they were used as a means of travel over deep snow during the long winters of Nordic countries. Early skiers used a single staff to aid in balance and to help control their speed on downhill descents. On flat and uphill terrain, they used the staff to push and glide forward on their skis. On downhill terrain, they would place the staff between their legs, much like a witch rides a broom, and by raising their hands and forcing the other end of the staff down into the snow, they could control their speed and create a braking action.

As skiing evolved from transportation to sport, skis got shorter and lighter, and skiers discovered that two poles could be used more efficiently for balance as well as for providing propulsion. When skiing further evolved into downhill and Nordic (or cross-country) forms of skiing, Nordic skiers quickly discovered that poles could play an important role by involving large upper-body muscles, thus adding significant power and speed to their skiing. It probably wasn't long before people realized that a pair of poles would also be much more efficient than a single walking stick for hiking, and "trekking poles" were born. Trekking poles have been popular with serious hikers and mountaineers for decades. They help hikers balance on rough terrain and take some of the load off legs while carrying heavy packs on a long climb or hike.

In the early 1900s, Nordic skiers began using poles to train and condition during the off-season. They would walk, run, or "bound" uphill on the same trails that would become ski trails with the coming of winter. In the 1970s, I began cross-country or Nordic skiing and soon after began using poles during the off-season to condition for winter competition. In 1984, while I was training for cross-country ski competition, it occurred to me that striding with poles was such a great form of exercise that it should not be limited to cross-training for skiers and other athletes. I realized that by adding a pair of rubber tips to poles, one could use them on city streets and sidewalks, as well as on trails, and that walkers and runners could turn their "half-body exercises" into total-body exercise with health and fitness benefits very similar to cross-country skiing. I soon discovered that, tempo for tempo, walking or running with poles was actually an even more effective exercise than was cross-country skiing. When one applies force to poles while cross-country skiing, there is significantly less resistance than when walking or running, because one is standing on skis, which are designed to glide as easily as possible.

Since then, only a small number of runners have taken an interest in using poles to increase the exercise benefits of their workouts, while walkers have been far more enthusiastic about the idea of using poles. Those for whom the ability to ambulate and remain independent was slipping away as a result of "normal" effects of aging have been among the most enthusiastic users of walking poles. People with osteoarthritis have found that using poles can decrease pain-causing stress on their hips, knees, and feet. Aging exercisers who were beginning to feel a lack of confidence due to declining overall muscle fitness and balance have found that a pair of poles not only gives them added balance and confidence but also rapidly improves overall muscle tone.

Walking poles have proven to be a very effective and useful rehabilitation device that can, in many cases, be used in lieu of canes, crutches, and walkers. At the other end of the fitness spectrum, the use of poles for sports training is no longer restricted to cross-country/Nordic athletes. Demanding, high-intensity total-body aerobic workout regimens have been designed and used successfully to simultaneously build overall muscle endurance and maximum aerobic fitness. These demanding workouts combine running, bounding, skipping, diagonal stride, and skate-ski simulation and "low-walking" to create a safe, highly efficient, and effective total-body workout. (More on that later.)

Walking poles are no longer just for hikers. They are among the simplest and most versatile fitness tools available. They can be used effectively throughout the entire spectrum of fitness building, from rehabilitation to high-performance training.

WALKING, HIKING, AND TREKKING POLES—WHAT'S THE DIFFERENCE?

The terms *hiking poles* and *trekking poles* can be used interchangeably when referring to modern, lightweight poles used in pairs. The terms *hiking* and *trekking* have essentially the same relationship as jogging and running. Hiking/trekking poles have been around for decades. (Note: Trekking poles are always used in pairs, while the term *hiking poles* can be applied to both single- and two-pole versions. Hiking poles can range in design from a handcrafted single walking pole, to a single cane-like pole, to a pair of lightweight, high-tech poles, which some call hiking poles and others refer to as trekking poles [i.e., jogging shoes vs. running shoes]. For this discussion, I will only describe hiking poles used as a pair.) Their primary purpose has been to help add balance on rough, unstable, or rocky terrain, take some of the stress off legs when carrying a heavy backpack on long hikes, and add power when ascending and braking when descending steep slopes. The poles are generally of a three-piece, tele-scoping design, which allows them to be compacted to a small size and attached to or stowed in a backpack when not in use. They are made of strong, light-weight aluminum tubing and have sharp, hardened or carbide steel tips designed to provide sure traction even on ice and in rocky streambeds. They also have "baskets" near the tips, designed to keep the tips from sinking deep into snow, streambeds, or mud.

Fitness walking poles are a newer development. In 1985, when I came up with the concept of using poles to create a new total-body exercise version of walking, I quickly realized that hardened steel tips were far from ideal for "urban fitness trekking." I designed the first long-wearing, shock-dampening rubber tips for walking poles, allowing trekking to make the move from the mountains and tundra to the city. I experimented with different types and designs of poles to find the right combination of strength, stiffness, lightness, and vibration dampening. I tried various types of aluminum, fiberglass, and graphite composite poles and found that only high-quality aluminum one-piece poles met strict performance requirements at an economical cost.

In 1997, Finnish ski pole manufacturer Exel became the next company to enter the walking pole market. Soon every manufacturer of ski poles in the world was offering a version of walking poles. Because of the rapid acceptance of walking poles throughout Scandinavia, walking poles are generally referred to as "Nordic" walking poles. Nordic walking poles are now available in one-piece designs with either lightweight aluminum or graphite composite shafts, as well as two- and three-piece telescoping poles made of aluminum, graphite composites, or combinations of graphite composites and aluminum.

The quality of walking poles runs a wide gamut. Unfortunately, many ski and trekking pole manufacturers have jumped on the Nordic/fitness walking bandwagon by just adding a pair of rubber tips to their existing ski and hiking poles. In Europe, the popularity of Nordic/fitness walking has grown to such proportions that one can even purchase a pair of low-priced, often poor-quality, poles at local groceries and gas stations.

So, what should one look for in purchasing Nordic/fitness walking poles? When it comes to both safety and function, the first criterion should be good vibration dampening. Vibration is a two-pronged problem when it comes to walking poles. Most importantly, vibration is an enemy of healthy connective tis-sue. "Tennis elbow" will soon have its walking pole counterpart in "Nordic walk-ing elbow," both because too many poles are being sold with poor vibration dampening characteristics and because many Nordic/fitness walkers are not getting adequate instruction in their use. Both aluminum and graphite compos-ite poles can provide good vibration dampening if designed and engineered properly. When it comes to two-and three-piece telescoping poles, the first sign of quality design and engineering is quietness. Poorly designed and engineered walking poles of any construction will be noisy and/or vibrate noticeably upon landing and will prove to be no bargain, no matter how low the price.

The next thing to look for is comfortable hand grips. Every pole manufacturer calls its grip "ergonomic." *Ergonomic* actually means "designed to reduce fatigue and discomfort." Most Nordic/fitness walking pole grips were originally designed for cross-country/Nordic or downhill/alpine ski poles. All of these grips come with either simple adjustable straps or sophisticated/complicated strapping systems with Velcro closures. Personally, I find straps to be uncomfortable by nature. While they are necessary for skiing and are less uncomfortable when used with a gloved hand, I contend that with a grip design that is truly ergonomic they are unnecessary for walking poles and are hot, chafing, and circulation-inhibiting, especially when used with bare hands in warm weather. Rather than just recycling an existing ski pole grip, I designed a strapless grip specifically to meet the demands of Nordic/fitness walking poles. Instead of relying on straps to maintain control of the poles without the need to hold the grips with clenched fists while applying force, I put a flare on the grips both above and below the hand so that any amount of force can be applied to the grip, and control of the pole can be maintained during the forward movement of the arm with a relaxed hand. In the event of a fall while using poles, my strapless design also significantly decreases the likelihood of any wrist injury. Just remember, simply calling anything ergonomic does not guarantee the reduction of fatigue and maximization of comfort. Try strapped and strapless poles, and decide for yourself which you prefer. A 15-degree positive-angle grip helps maintain a healthy neutral wrist position. This positive angle can be achieved by angling the grip forward or an angled flare on the rear of the grip.

Another major thing to look for is impact protection. You'll land walking poles 1,700 to 2,000 times on surfaces that can range from soft grass to concrete. Impact shock/trauma can be even more damaging to the body than vibration. Shock absorption in poles can range from sophisticated steel spring and elastomer antishock designs to simple rubber tips. In my opinion, the most effective impact prevention comes from learning to use poles properly. Even the most sophisticated antishock mechanisms will not protect a person who does not learn how to use poles properly. While "antishock systems" can be attractive marketing features, they can wear out and provide a false sense of safety to those who are offered little or no instruction in the safe and proper use of walking poles. Soft, cushioning, long-wearing rubber tips *along with proper technique* are the best long-term solution.

Speaking of technique, the last thing to consider in choosing a Nordic/fitness walking pole is the kind of instructions that come along with the poles. Depending on the brand, instructions for use can range from nonexistent to a comprehensive user's manual and instructional video. To get the best results and safety out of using walking poles, you'll need more in the way of instruction than you'll find in this chapter. Look for poles that include clear, detailed, and comprehensive instructional materials, or count on hiring a certified instructor if you want to get the most out of walking with poles.

Sizing the Poles

To select a walking pole of the correct height, place the tip of the pole even with your heel, and hold the hand grip in your hand. When your upper arm is perpendicular to the ground, your forearm should be roughly parallel to the ground. This length generally will be approximately equal to your height multiplied by 0.70 to 0.75.

Fitness Walking with Poles

Since 1985, when I first conceived of the idea of making walking with poles a viable form of regular total-body exercise, the activity has experienced a steady growth in popularity. I called this new form of total-body exercise "exerstriding," because this new way of walking provided an effective way to exercise nearly every major muscle while striding (whether walking, running, bounding, or skipping). When a ski pole manufacturer introduced the concept to Finnish walkers in 1997, they called it "Nordic walking," and in just a few years it became the fastest growing fitness trend across Europe. Because of the explosive growth in popularity of fitness walking with poles in Europe, Nordic walking has become the widely accepted generic term for the activity. Exerstriding is simply the original form of Nordic walking. My techniques differ somewhat from the Nordic walking techniques that are currently being promoted in Europe. I've tried every suggested technique of fitness walking with poles and remain convinced my Exerstride Method Nordic walking techniques are both the safest and most effective, so my discussion of fitness walking with poles will be based on my many years of experience and results of studies done with Exerstride Method fitness walking with poles (or exerstriding).

Why have so many walkers in the United States and around the world converted to fitness walking with poles? The easiest way to understand the rapidly rising popularity of using poles while walking is to get a feel for how it changes the nature of walking and makes it a genuine total-body exercise.

Try this simple demonstration, which will give you a real feel for just how this new exercise form can involve so many important muscles in the upper body. While seated at a desk or table, extend both arms out as if offering a friendly handshake. Now make a fist with both hands and place your fists on the surface of the table with your thumbs up. Next, push one fist, then the other, alternately on the surface. Note how muscles in your trunk, arms, shoulder, chest, and back contract each time you push on the surface of the table. While the muscle contractions that occur in this demonstration are isometric (since the arms do not move during the demonstration), 1,700 to 2,000 similar isokinetic contractions occur each mile when one walks with poles.

THE BENEFITS OF WALKING WITH POLES

There are many additional health and fitness benefits that can be enjoyed by walkers who choose to add walking poles to their favorite exercise.

In a study published in the *American College of Sports Medicine Journal* in 1995, women who began walking with poles immediately burned an average of more than 23 percent more calories—without feeling any change in perceived exertion. (By intentionally increasing the level of exertion of the upper-body muscles involved, metabolic increases of up to 78 percent have been recorded.) It should be noted that more than 50 percent of one's muscle mass is in the upper body, and as this large amount of muscle mass is recruited to help move the body, one can expend significantly more energy, yet actually feel as though one is doing less work since the work is shared by many more large muscles. I call that working out smarter rather than working out harder.

During another 12-week study in 1992, women walked with poles 4 days per week for 30 to 45 minutes. At the beginning and end of the 12-week period they were tested for upper-body muscle endurance. They recorded a 38 percent increase in muscle endurance at the end of the study.

Besides increasing calorie burn and muscle endurance, the addition of a large amount of upper-body muscle mass to walking results in other health and fitness benefits. Pulse rate will increase ten to fifteen beats per minute from just walking at the same pace. Because part of the body's weight is supported by the upper body as one pushes on the pole, the impact forces to hips, knees, and feet can be decreased by up to 26 percent. For those who suffer from lower-body joint pain resulting from osteoarthritis, walking with poles can in many cases remove a sufficient amount of stress from lower-body joints to allow pain-free walking. Because part of one's body weight is supported by the upper-body when using poles, the weight-bearing work done by the upper-body musculoskeletal system may also play an important role in helping to preserve upper-body bone density. For those who have balance or posture problems, most find that walking with poles helps improve both.

Walking with poles has both psychological and neurological benefits as well. A study conducted at the University of Wisconsin–LaCrosse looked at the psychological profiles of eighty-seven previously sedentary women between the ages of 20 and 50. They were all tested before and after the completion of the 12-week study. During the study, twenty-nine women simply walked, and thirty others walked with poles 30 to 45 minutes per day, 4 days per week; another twenty-eight remained inactive as a control group for the same period of time. A standardized "Profile of Mood States" and "Total Body Cathexis" assessment was used to gauge the effects. There were no significant differences over the period of the study among the control group. Those who walked with poles showed significant improvements in levels of depression, anger, vigor, fatigue, total mood disturbances, and total body cathexis. In contrast, those who just walked showed significant improvement in only vigor and total body cathexis. It was speculated that use of the poles may have resulted in increased production of endorphins. These naturally produced opiate-like neurotransmitters interact with the opiate receptors in the brain to reduce our perception of pain, having a similar action to drugs such as morphine and codeine. In addition to decreased feelings of pain, secretion of endorphins can lead to feelings of euphoria, modulation of appetite, release of sex hormones, and enhancement of the immune response. With high endorphin levels, we feel less pain and fewer negative effects of stress

In addition, cross-patterning exercises have been demonstrated to increase levels of dopamine in the body. Dopamine is another neurotransmitter that facilitates critical brain function and can lessen levels of depression. Finally, studies on the effect of Nordic skiing on neurological functioning done in Scandinavia demonstrated improved neurologic functioning. This may have been the result of the cross-pattern nature of the exercise or simply the stimulation of neurologic function that occurs as a result of continuous, rhythmic contractions of the trunk and back muscle, which stimulate the flow of cerebral spinal fluid and may improve overall nervous system function. While there is still much to be learned about the exact nature and cause of neurologic outcome, it's common for walkers to report "feeling better" in ways apart from physical when they begin walking with poles.

One might ask, If walking with poles has all of these advantages, why isn't everyone walking with poles? The answer to this question is probably part psychosocial and part cultural. In the United States, fitness walking with poles has encountered resistance. While we Americans may love to identify with trends and fashion, most of us are equally averse to being the first on our block to do, buy, or use anything until it is a bona fide trend. In Europe, fitness walking with poles has been quickly embraced, and the activity has experienced an explosive growth in popularity in just seven years. We'll leave the reasons for this phenomenon to the psychologists and sociologists to explain, but needless to say, once fitness walking with poles achieves "trend status" in the United States, it is very likely that a rapidly increasing number of people who walk for fitness will likely be doing so with poles.

How to Use Walking Poles

Whether one uses poles for prevention or rehabilitation of injury, to build overall "functional" fitness, or as a training tool for improving athletic performance, the basic technique is the same.

START WITH A "HANDSHAKE"

Exerstriding is easy to learn. If you can walk, you can learn to exerstride in just minutes. In terms of how the arms and legs move, walking and exerstriding are very similar. The only difference is in the range of movement (ROM) of the arms. When walking and when exerstriding, the arms move in opposition to the legs. That is, when the right leg moves forward, the left arm moves forward and vice versa. This is called diagonal striding (as in cross-country skiing) or cross-crawl or cross-patterning. You do not have to think about it when you walk, and you will not have to think about it when you exerstride. It will happen automatically (if you allow it to). It's the way our bodies are programmed to move.

When one walks, the arms move in front of the body as they swing forward and behind the body as they swing backward (see Figure 2) When you Exerstride, the arms will move farther in front of the body. The arm is raised into what I call the "handshake position." The arm is extended as though you are offering it for a friendly, confident handshake. Do not lock the elbow so that the arm is completely straight. There should be a slight, comfortable bend in the arm at the elbow. (This "handshake position" is the first key to maximizing the benefits of exerstriding. I'll explain why later.) Since the arm is extended farther out in front of the body than it is when walking, the arm does not travel as far rearward on the back swing. In fact, the arm will only travel back far enough to roughly align with the upper portion of the opposite leg as it moves forward (see Figure 3) In both walking and exerstriding, the arm moves in a pendulum-like motion, with the shoulder joint being the pivot point. Note the difference in the ROM in Figure 4.

Figure 2

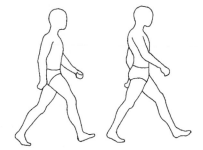

Figure 3

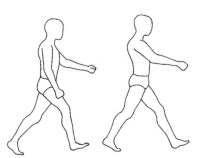

Figure 4

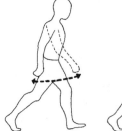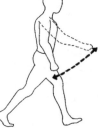

If you remember that the ROM of the arms is the only major difference between walking and exerstriding, you'll be able to learn in just minutes. Unfortunately, some of those who pick up a pair of walking poles for the first time (especially cerebral types) refuse to believe that it could actually be so easy to learn. They kick their brains into high gear and try to analyze the fairly complex biomechanics of walking. As they try to intellectualize something that is actually second nature, the results are usually disastrous, or at the very least frustrating. If we all believed that it was necessary to think ourselves through the act of walking, we'd probably all be reading and writing before we learned to walk! So as you learn to exerstride, give your mind a rest and let the body do what comes naturally.

Begin by holding the pole grips loosely in your hands, with your arms hanging completely relaxed at your sides. The tips of the poles should rest on the ground behind you. Relax your hands, and hold on to the poles just tightly enough to keep them in your hands. You do not ever need to maintain a tight grip on the poles. Simply begin to walk, and walk until you are walking in a normal, comfortable stride, with your arms swinging slightly in front and then behind your body with each stride. (The more you think, the harder it will be!) At first you'll simply allow the pole tips to drag along the ground. You won't need anyone to tell you when you've gotten to a normal walking stride. You'll recognize it—you've been doing it for years. If you find that your mind has kicked into high gear and as a result you simply can't get into a normal walking stride, simply stop and begin again until your mind disengages from the task and you begin to walk with a normal, relaxed stride. Then simply begin to extend your arms a little farther forward with each stride until you have extended them into the handshake position with each stride. If, as you work at extending the arm with each stride, you lose coordination between the arms and the legs and just can't maintain a natural coordination, stop and begin again. Try what I call the "kick-start" technique: Begin by extending one leg (whichever one you like) in front of the other as though you are taking a comfortable, normal stride. Then extend the opposite arm in front in the handshake position. The arm on the same side as the leading leg should hang loosely at your side. From this position, simply lean back and push off the back leg and you'll "kick-start" the motion. The opposite arm will automatically swing forward, and if you push down with the extended arm, you will begin with perfect coordination of the arms and legs. If your arms and legs get out of sync, just stop and initiate the kick-start technique again.

If you've tried the kick-start technique and you're still having trouble coordinating the movement of the arms and legs, don't allow yourself to get discouraged. I've taught thousands of people to walk with poles, and I've never met anyone yet who could not learn the basics in 30 minutes or less. Just hang in there! The final instructional trick I pull out of my bag is called the "march technique." This technique relies on the fact that when proper technique is achieved, each foot will land at the same time as the tip of the pole held in the opposite hand. A march tune can be used to establish a strong beat that co-incides with the landing of the feet. Somehow tying this strong audio cue with the footfall facilitates a corresponding landing of the pole on the same beat. I've taught many people to exerstride who were convinced that they were too unco-ordinated to ever learn. The march technique is usually what allowed them to learn when all else failed. In addition to providing a beat on the landing of the foot and opposite tip, the march technique provides an important distraction for those of you who might still insist that the only way you can learn anything is to think it through. Exerstriding really is as easy and as natural as walking.

Once you are able to simply walk and extend your arm into the handshake position with each stride, you will feel the tip of the pole land and create a resistance to the rearward swing of the arm. Once you've got your arm and leg movement coordinated, push against that resistance, and you have begun to exerstride.

Remember, don't grip the pole tightly, and don't attempt to control where the tip lands. You do not lift the poles and place the tips. You simply raise your arm into the handshake position. As the arms swing forward like a pendulum into the handshake position, the tips will automatically land in the "right" place, and the pole will contact the ground at the "correct" (not 90-degree) angle. If you maintain a very light grip on the poles as you swing them forward, the tips will automatically lift off the ground and come to a landing in just the right place. *Always attempt to land the tip as lightly as possible, and once it makes contact, only then should you attempt to apply as much force as possible* to the pole. Initially, you may have some difficulty with bouncing and slip-ping of the tips as they land. At first, you will find that your dominant hand will be much more proficient in controlling the pole and tip than is your nondomi-nant hand. Very quickly you will develop improved coordination with both hands, and you'll also develop the timing of your push so that you'll get a good grip on the surface with your tip with every stride. Be patient with yourself. It will take a couple of days or weeks until you feel completely relaxed and at ease when exerstriding, but very soon it will become as automatic and effortless as walking.

THE ARM MOVEMENT SHOULD RESEMBLE A PUMP HANDLE

As you learn to exerstride you will probably tend to keep your upper arms fairly still, unless you pay special attention to developing proper/more effective tech-nique. Without instruction and attention, most people will tend to push the poles by opening and closing the elbow joint instead of by pumping the entire arm in a pendulum-like motion. (This is more like the Euro-Nordic walking technique, which I believe to be far less effective.) Remember that the arm should actually serve as a lever that transfers the major work of exerstriding to the large muscles of the trunk. The arm should keep a fixed shape, with just a slight bend in the elbow, and should move while pivoting from the shoulder. If you've ever operated an old-fashioned water pump, you should see the similarity between the motion of the arm and the action of the handle on the pump. Keep this image of the arm moving like a pump handle in your mind, then remember to extend your arm into the handshake position with each stride, and you will develop an expert, highly effective technique in no time. The greater attention you give to developing good technique, the more overall benefits you will derive from every step you take with walking poles.

As in cross-country skiing, the arms and legs should move with a smooth, rhythmic cadence. Your stride should be just like your normal, relaxed walking stride. As you push with your upper body to help you move forward, there is often a tendency to lengthen the stride, so pay special attention to maintaining a normal stride length. Attempt to make your entire motion as fluid as possible. With proper arm action, the large muscles in the trunk will do most of the work. If you feel your triceps tiring quickly when you walk with poles, you're probably not moving your arms properly. As you exerstride, you should be able to see your upper arms moving forward and back. If you glance down and your forearms are moving but your upper arms are relatively still, it's time to remember the handshake and the pump handle arm motion. When you use your arms correctly, you actually get the maximum overall muscle mass involved. The more force you apply, the greater the intensity of the contractions of all of the upper-body muscles involved. The more muscle mass that is involved in exercise, the higher the overall muscle and skeletal benefits, the higher the metabolic rate (more calories burned), the higher the level of cardiovascular development, and the less stress placed on any one muscle or joint. When you begin to fitness walk with poles, many muscles may be quite deconditioned and have little endurance, but since the involved muscles do 1,700 to 2,000 contractions per mile, they will rapidly increase in endurance and, over time, in strength.

Hiking and Trekking with Poles

For years, hikers and trekkers have been using poles without the benefit of any significant instruction. For the most part they have relied on instinct. Generally, for hiking on trails the poles were adjusted so that when the arms were bent at 90 degrees and the forearm was parallel to the ground the pole would address the ground at a 90-degree angle. This allowed hikers to use the poles to provide additional balance and take some weight off their legs. The poles were only used to add power and help propel the body when making ascents. Serious trekkers, like those who trek across miles of frozen tundra or polar regions pulling sleds filled with heavy supplies, soon discovered how important poles were in providing the total power to pull these heavy sleds over great distances.

The telescoping feature of hiking/trekking poles is especially important, given the extreme terrain often encountered by hikers and trekkers. First of all, there are some terrain and surface conditions where the use of poles proves to be impractical or impossible. Extremely steep ascents often require hikers and trekkers to use their hands and arms to pull themselves up steep rocky trails or faces. In these circumstances, telescoping poles can be stowed in, or attached to, backpacks until these difficult sections of trail are negotiated. Extreme descents may also require them to use their hands and arms to use basic climbing techniques to safely descend.

On long traverses where the hill slopes steeply up and down on each side of a very narrow trail, the uphill pole can be shortened slightly and the downhill pole lengthened to compensate for the terrain. On long, steep uphill trails, the poles can be slightly shortened to compensate for the steep terrain.

It is common for hikers and trekkers to lengthen their poles when making descents on a trail. The theory is that by placing the tips in front of the body, one can control the rate of descent by using the poles to create a braking action. I consider this technique to be very risky. Placing the poles ahead of the body on a descent means that the poles will address the slope at a low angle. The steeper the descent, the lower the angle at which the poles will contact the ground. This creates the possibility that a pole plant could fail to provide the desired braking effect and could even lead to a dangerous face-first fall forward. Instead, I recommend that the poles not be adjusted on downhill descents. Rather than placing the pole tips in front of the body, they should be placed behind the body at a maximum stabilizing 90-degree angle to the slope of the hill. Then bend the knees slightly and sit back into the hill a bit while supporting your weight with the poles. This will lower your center of gravity and create four points of firm contact with the hill. In a worst case scenario you will fall a much shorter distance back into the hill and on a much more padded part of your anatomy.

USING WALKING POLES FOR DISEASE AND INJURY PREVENTION AND REHABILITATION

In recent years, obesity and diabetes have replaced smoking as the leading health risks. Walking with poles has proven to be a very useful tool in treating and preventing both of these health risks. It can help those with borderline type 2 diabetes more effectively control their blood sugar levels, as exercising muscles are more sensitive to insulin. One study showed the risk of developing diabetes was reduced by 24 percent by the expenditure of 2,000 calories per week through exercise. A person who would burn 1,600 calories per week by walking would, on average, burn around 2,000 calories in the same time with no change in perceived exertion.

Walking with poles also helps build overall muscle mass, burns more calories, and takes significant stress off the lower joints of obese walkers. This can help walkers increase overall metabolic rates, and remain more motivated by accelerated weight loss and exercise for greater durations, thereby improving results. Often, the greatest challenge facing obese persons wishing to begin a regular program of exercise is that even walking can be difficult and painful. By taking significant pressure off hips, knees, and feet by using poles and by recruiting latent upper-body strength through the use of the poles, many are not only able to walk greater distances and durations, but they also burn more calories and begin to more effectively increase overall metabolism.

Walking poles are being used in cardiac rehabilitation programs. Many cardiac rehab patients are able to more easily achieve their prescribed target heart rates without running. Poles also are being used in exercise programs aimed at maintaining overall bone density through total-body weight-bearing exercise. Others use the poles to strengthen back muscles and stabilize lumbar spines and shoulder joints. Poles can help mobilize osteoarthritic patients and thus improve health and function of joints. Putting joints to regular good use can help to preserve the health of the joint following joint replacement surgery.

Two research studies conducted at Hines Veterans Administration Hospital in Illinois showed that subjects with peripheral vascular disease and Parkinson's disease both benefited from using walking poles for exercise. The use of poles improved both balance and tolerance to exercise in both groups and by doing so improved subjects' quality of life.

Walking poles provide both practical and psychosocial advantages versus canes, crutches, and walkers in many clinical applications. The scope of application of walking with poles as a preventative and rehab tool is expanding as more health professionals learn of the tool and come up with more and more creative applications.

Perhaps the greatest preventative role that walking poles has to play will be in terms of making the health and fitness benefits of regular exercise both more accessible and attractive to populations that have found other common exercise prescriptions impossible to adhere to. Walking with poles combines effective aerobic exercise with total-body muscle conditioning and can be done by persons of any age, at any fitness level, and at any intensity, and still realize motivating results.

Moving Beyond the "No Pain, No Gain" Paradigm

When I first began to walk with poles, there were serious questions in my mind concerning the relative benefits compared with the many types of exercise I had employed in the past. Having come from a competitive athletic background, I still believed the common dictum "No pain, no gain." For years I had routinely exercised through pain in an effort to enhance my athletic performance. When I began to use poles, suddenly I was exercising totally without pain and strain. Since 1985, my workouts have consisted of walking with poles at generally less than 50 percent of my maximum age-predicted heart rate. I barely raise a sweat (I perspire only enough to create a cooling effect). I haven't huffed or panted during exercise for years. For a long time I hardly felt like I was even "exercising" until one day I opened my *Webster's* dictionary and looked up the word. According to *Webster's*, *exercise* is "an act of putting to use." I realized that what exerstriding had done for me was to allow me to simultaneously put my entire body to good use with a single exercise. I now believe that one of the main reasons so few people participate in any program of regular physical exercise is because too much of what most experts prescribe as "exercise" puts the body to abuse rather than simply putting it to use. Most fitness experts base their exercise prescriptions on exercises designed for athletes. Most of these prescriptions were designed specifically to improve athletic performance. Many of these prescriptions, while certainly capable of improving the physical performance of athletes, quite simply put the bodies of ordinary people to abuse. For the vast majority of exercisers who are not competitive athletes, and thus not interested in abusing their bodies in a quest for a higher level of performance, these prescriptions likely do more harm than good. This ill-advised vision of "exercise" has actually turned millions of people off to leading more active lives. Most people just want to feel better, have at least somewhat slimmer, healthier bodies, have more energy, and function better. While certain exerstriding techniques can be used to enhance physical performance, exerstriding is a great way to put the entire body to good use and in doing so to improve the way we look, feel, and function.

Summary

While exercises that increase muscle strength and mass have been shown to be essential to enhancing athletic performance, what is functionally important is establishing an acceptable baseline level of muscle strength and then putting the body to use in ways that increase muscle endurance. Fitness walking with poles simultaneously improves aerobic, muscle, joint, bone, and lymph function. The synergistic nature of fitness walking with poles makes it an extremely efficient means to accomplish more in less time, with little risk of injury and maximum benefits to an individual's physical function.

Tom Rutlin is president of Exerstrider Fitness in Madison, Wisconsin. He pioneered the use of poles to build total body fitness and improve general health and has been walking with poles for more than twenty years.

Prevention of Climbing Injuries in Hiking, Rock Climbing, and Mountaineering

by John Loleit

Hiking, rock climbing, and mountaineering, whether near or far, demand that you prepare yourself adequately. Your enjoyment of outdoor environments is related to your forethought and preparedness to maintain mental and physical comfort.

This section is dedicated to preparing you for and refreshing your common sense and providing some solutions and ideas for your comfort. You are your own life support. Even a short hike with simple problems can turn out to be traumatic, so be ready!

Preparing for Your Hike

KNOW YOUR LIMITATIONS

Your physical conditioning is the key factor in making your hike or mountain climb enjoyable. For anyone over the age of 40, a phsycian's OK is a good idea before starting out. Taking on a hike that will overtax your abilities is destined to spell disaster. You want to feel good after the hike so that you have energy to spare in case you need it. While on the trail, take at least one 10-minute break each hour and a 30-minute break if you are normally an inactive person. Find shade, sit down, and elevate your feet. Do not remove your boots or shoes because your feet, as well as your hands, naturally swell when hiking. Putting your boots back on could be uncomfortable.

BE FAMILIAR WITH THE TRAIL YOU ARE HIKING

The terrain, weather, trail surface condition, elevation, grade, and slope can help you decide how your trip will proceed.

Trails are simply rated: Easy trails require little physical challenge; they are smooth, level, and wide. Moderate trails offer more physical challenge over some steep terrain. The trail surface contains rocks and roots that make for some unstable footing. Difficult trails require a high degree of skill and offer greater physical challenge. A better indicator for trail difficulty is the time involved in elevation gain. Use the gauge of at least 1 hour per 1,000 feet of elevation gain or loss. Hiking downhill is not necessarily easier. Your time will vary depending on your own pace and physical condition.

Trail maps and guides can be obtained from outdoor recreation stores, land management agencies, trailheads, and the Internet. Be sure to review the map and apply it to your own capabilities. Mountain passes, steep terrain, water crossings, swamps, and high and low elevations all have an impact on how long a trail will take to hike. Try to go with someone who has done the trail before.

TUNE INTO THE WEATHER FORECAST

Before there was weather radio and television, many people understood the progression of weather and development because they took the time to look up and around. Today's weather satellites and television coverage can be extremely helpful in providing an accurate forecast. If you are planning a mountain climb, take note that weather changes are less predictable at higher elevations. Temperatures can easily drop 3° to 5° for every 1,000 feet you climb. Wind is a factor that is frequently overlooked; it can drain you of energy and heat in cold environments and dehydrate you in hot environments. Extreme temperature swings can happen after storms or in the desert when the sun sets.

Take time throughout the climb to look around and observe the clouds and any changes in wind direction. If you are traveling in low areas or washes, remember it doesn't have to be raining where you are for a flash flood to develop. While walking downhill or downstream, frequently look behind you for dark rain clouds building up, which potentially could develop into a flash flood. As little as 6 inches of rushing water can knock you off your feet.

Lightning occurs in all thunderstorms. Taking shelter under trees, near utility lines, in low areas, or inside small caves is dangerous. If caught in the open, drop into a low squat, with your head between your knees, and place a tarp or sleeping pad under your feet for insulation. To calculate how far the thunderstorm is from you, count the number of seconds between a flash of lightning and the next clap of thunder. Divide this number by 5 to determine the distance to the lightning in miles. Never underestimate the power or threat of thunderstorms.

TELL SOMEONE WHERE YOU ARE GOING

Telling someone or leaving a note is the most important thing to do before you set out on your hike. Tell someone where you are going; who you might be going with; possible delays that could be encountered, the make, model, and license number of the car you will be in; and when you can be expected back. Some trails and climbs have mandatory sign-in and -out systems, and many have a volunteer registration system set up at the trailhead of your hike, so be sure to sign in. Also, remember to sign out when you return, so there is an indication that you have been there and returned. Do not leave a note on your car that could tell anyone passing by how long you will be gone or when you will return.

The second most important thing you do is to stick to the plan. Deciding during your hike to take another trail or any diversion from the original plan will increase the time necessary to find or help you should you need assistance. No one but you knew you made the decision to change from the original plans.

When you return, let the person you told know that you have arrived back safely.

PREHIKE AND MOUNTAIN CLIMB MEAL

The prehike and mountain climb meal may be the most important one you have all day. Take the opportunity to eat and drink to give you the energy needed in the beginning stages of the hike. If you are accustomed to little more than a cup of coffee for breakfast, you will be running on empty before you get started. Caffeinated drinks should be kept to a minimum, as they are diuretics and can set the stage for dehydration later down the trail. Keep in mind that starting a climb with a full reserve of food and water will make the hike more pleasant. All too often hikers begin already behind in their food and liquid intake. Don't wait to start drinking water on the climb; you should be fully hydrated before you start. Eating foods high in carbohydrates will best provide energy for the extended hike. Cereal, fruit, and juice are best, and keep foods high in fat to a minimum because they require more energy to digest, which reduces energy available for the hike.

WHAT TO WEAR

Dress appropriately for the predicted weather conditions, and be prepared for the potential weather changes that could happen at any time during an outing. Standard attire begins with a hat that can keep you warm or cool and block the sun. Heat rises from your body, and much of it is lost through your head. During hot weather a hat actually keeps you cooler by keeping the direct sun off your head. In a cold environment it holds in heat escaping from your head, which in turn can keep your feet warm. A bandanna should be standard on any hiking or climbing trip. It has multiple uses including as a sling, bandage, towel, or napkin.

Dressing in layers will allow moisture to wick away from the skin and gives you numerous heating and cooling options. Avoid cotton clothing, because it keeps moisture closer to your skin, takes longer to dry, and retains no heat when wet. Polypropylene, Capilene, Thermax, Coolmax, wool, or any material that wicks moisture away from the body will keep you comfortable in all seasons. Your feet may be the last you think of, but they do the most work for you. A small blister can make the difference between a good or bad hike. The same materials suggested for your clothing also apply to the socks that you wear.

Climbing shoes and hiking boots should have the support that you need for ankles and or arches, but more importantly a good sturdy tread. Tennis shoes, court shoes, and walking shoes may not have the sole that is needed to give your foot stability on the trail. Climbing shoes and hiking boots are designed for use on a trail or rough mountain terrain.

EQUIPMENT YOU'LL NEED/WHAT TO PACK

The length of the hike, whether the hike is in the desert or mountains, and how long you plan to be gone will dictate the type of equipment and necessities you'll need to take along. You can customize the items needed based on your personal preference, and always be prepared for the unexpected. If the hike takes longer than expected or you have experienced trouble along the way, the essential items in your pack will help develop and maintain your comfort zone. Take items that can have multiple uses.

There are a number of popular gadgets and specialized equipment that can help today's hiker and mountaineer. The wrong jacket or sophisticated electronic equipment can be a burden or a frustration. The key is to know how to use them to suit your needs.

Following is a list of basic items to pack.

Trail map, guidebook, GPS unit, and/or topographic map and compass. Trail maps usually are confined to the specific trail you wish to take and may suffice, especially if it is a popular and heavily used trail. Guidebooks provide more detail of the natural and cultural history of the trail and possibly specific points of interest and landmarks as well. Topographic maps go beyond the narrow boundaries of the trail, so in the case of your losing the trail, this type of map will provide more landmarks than the other maps. In today's high-tech world, the global positioning system (GPS) is the latest gadget to have. It will keep track of your location through the use of satellites. Learn to use it before embarking on your climb, and take extra batteries.

Water. Water is the most essential item to always have with you on any hike or climb, in any climate, under any circumstance. Water is brain power and affects everything that you do. Without it, or limited amounts of it, the body starts to shut down to conserve what it has left. Therefore, never ration your water. Drink often and to quench your thirst. A highly functional brain that is not deprived of water will help you make the right decisions at the time you need to make them. Sports drinks that contain electrolytes replace the minerals and essential nutrients that you have sweated out of your system. They provide some energy and keep you going. Remember to drink plenty of fluids during mountain climbs that are in cold environments, because fully hydrated climbers stay much warmer.

Food and snacks. The length and difficulty of the hike will dictate the kinds and types of foods to carry along. Small, frequent portions will provide a constant source of energy throughout the day. There are long-term energy foods, like pasta, breads, potatoes, and vegetables, and short-term energy foods, like fresh and dried fruits, that keep your energy levels up throughout the hike. A diet that contains fruits, nuts, jerky, cheese, granola, energy bars, pretzels, and even candy will add variety and energy for your hike. During the day, major portions should be of carbohydrates, while larger quantities of proteins and fats consumed at the evening meal will help prime you for the challenges of the next day.

Extra clothing. Depending on the weather forecast, plan for the unexpected to happen. Waterproof or water-repellent clothing is light and compactable and can provide the added protection and/or warmth you'll need to maintain your comfort level. A hat should almost always be worn to protect you from the sun or to keep your head dry and warm. A bandanna has a variety of uses, and always carry an extra pair of socks for longer hikes. Carry enough extra clothing to survive an overnight stay.

Fire starter/matches. With precautions to environmental and wildfire conditions, a campfire—or even a candle—can provide extreme comfort and keep you warm should you become lost. Smoke can be a signal to others in the area that you may be experiencing difficulty.

Army knife. A Boy Scout or Swiss Army knife, with extras such as tweezers and scissors, can come in very handy for a variety of needs. A sharp blade will help to reduce the number of injuries you have while cutting anything from rope to fruit.

First-aid Kit. Your personalized kit should contain some pain-relief medicine, prescriptions, self-adhesive bandages, moleskin, gauze, antiseptic, antibacterial or iodine wipes, instant ice packs, tweezers, sunscreen, sting and bite medications, and a small first-aid booklet.

Flashlight and batteries. A flashlight or headlamp can make setting up camp easier. If there were delays in the hike and darkness is closing in, light for the last part of the trail could prevent stumbles and keep you on the trail.

Cell phone and radio. Depending on where and how far from civilization you are, bring your cell phone. In case there is an emergency, the signal could be strong enough to make a connection. The more urbanized we get, cell phone towers may be able to pick up your signal for help. A compact radio can be very helpful if you become lost, as it will give updates on the weather and possible search progress. Listening to a radio, or CD player with a headset while hiking is highly discouraged. This reduces your ability to hear what is going on around you that could be as ominous as the warning buzz of a rattlesnake, the beautiful song of a bird, or the roar of an avalanche.

Whistle and bell. A whistle, on a lanyard around your neck, can be heard over greater distances than your shouts. Three short blasts are regarded as an emergency signal. If you are hiking or mountain climbing in areas where large animals live, a bell can be worn on the outside of your pack. The jingling of the bell will warn animals long in advance of your approach, thus avoiding startling any animals that may be about.

Emergency blanket. These inexpensive silver foil–like blankets are small, compact, and can be used as a shelter, poncho and blanket. Their reflective qualities make them a valuable tool to signal for help.

Hiking Poles. Hiking poles have started to replace the common hiking stick as a practical addition to your hiking and mountain-climbing equipment list. They can add rhythm and balance to your stride, reduce stress and strain on your joints, help you cross a stream, or measure the depth of snow.

Survival Tips

If you have become lost, at the very moment you realize this, *stop.* Traveling farther and thinking you know where to go may get you more disoriented and lost and therefore harder to find. *Do not panic.* Let your brain do the walking before you do. Maintaining a positive mental attitude will see a successful outcome to your dilemma.

Be alert to the three conditions that pose an immediate threat to your life: hyperthermia, dehydration, and hypothermia.

It cannot be stressed enough how important water is to your well-being. When the brain is stressed from lack of sufficient water, it loses its ability to function rationally. The muscles are not far behind. That is when mistakes are made that could lead to bigger problems later on. Do not ration your water. Drink frequently, even if you don't feel thirsty, and drink to quench your thirst no matter if it is a long distance before the next water source. The correct decisions you make now may save you later. To reduce moisture loss, stop talking, do not eat salty foods, and breathe through your nose.

A cell phone can be a lifesaver. Try your phone just in case it might work. Some phones have a GPS tracking system built into them, and the location of the call can be traced. Blowing your whistle three times in a row is a signal for emergency.

In hot weather, the ground could be 30° warmer than the air temperature. In cold climates, the ground or rock will rob you of heat.

Look through your pack and think what items can perform double duties, such as the reflective properties of an emergency blanket. Knowing that you have told someone where you were going, you stuck to your plan, and you're prepared helps with your anxiety and will eventually get you found.

Hiking Etiquette

- "Leave only footprints, take only photographs" has been a motto for a long time. Consider the consequences of picking one flower or taking a small cultural artifact. Multiply that by everyone who passes by, and you are left with nothing. You may be out on the trail alone but your act affects everyone. Others can no longer enjoy the beauty or wonder that struck you about the flower or artifact if you do choose to take it.

- Keep to the right as you hike on the trail. Be aware of hikers behind you who may be on a faster pace; let them pass. Limit walking side by side on a narrow trail to reduce the sudden approach of another hiker trying to pass. Walking near the trail's edge can also increase erosion and widen the trail.

- Stay on the trail. Cutting trail or making shortcuts increases erosion, defaces the natural beauty, and impacts both plants and animals.

- Keep your voice low to minimize the impact to other hikers and to increase your chances of seeing wildlife. Walk softly.

- Pack it in, pack it out. Reduce prepackaged food you plan to take with you, and place it in zip-lock bags, which can be used later to pack trash. The food carried this way is much lighter and easier to haul out.

- The need to "go." Everyone has to sooner or later. Some simple rules to follow: Be at least 200 feet from the trail or any water source. A small hole in the top 6 inches of soil is the most active to help break down material. Put any paper into a zip-lock bag, and double bag if necessary.

- Plant and animal etiquette. Staying on the trail will not impact fragile vegetation that reduces soil erosion and food or cover for wildlife. Learn the natural history of the plants and animals along the trail for better appreciation and understanding of their existence. Don't feed the wildlife. This upsets their natural cycle of nutrition and creates dependence on humans, is ecologically unsound, and reduces their fear of humans. When observing wildlife, no matter how adorable, beautiful, docile, or harmless they look, they are wild. Enjoy them from a distance.

Summary

Over the last few hundred years, the human race has evolved from primarily living outside to living inside. We now can control the climate of our homes, have water at the turn of a faucet, and have enough food stored in refrigerators that we don't have to deal with being outside. It is ironic that today we have to educate ourselves on how to behave and survive in the great outdoors. This chapter is to inspire your use of common sense, being prepared for the unexpected circumstances that occur, and maintaining a positive attitude. Using all three of these concepts will make your hiking, rock climbing, or mountaineering experience rewarding, challenging, and invigorating. So, go outside and hike a trail or climb a mountain!

John Loleit is employed by the City of Scottsdale Parks and Recreation Department as park coordinator for Pinnacle Peak Park and Trail. Previously, he served for 21 years as a park ranger for the National Park Service. Loleit lives in Glendale, Arizona, with his wife and son.

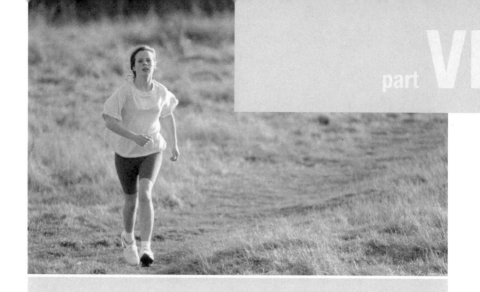

orthopedic surgery and podiatry management of outdoor recreational injuries

Parts III through V focused on specific injuries, rehabilitation, and prevention of reinjury. It is now time to look at your last treatment option—surgery. It should be stressed that surgery should only be used after failure of conservative therapy. Of course, there are emergency situations, such as displaced fractures and dislocations that need immediate surgery. Before you consider the surgical option, be sure you understand the risks of surgery and the rare possibility that you could actually be worse after surgery than better. Before you sign the surgical consent form, be sure that you understand the risks and rewards of surgery.

In this current era of medicine and surgery, specialization is rather common. In orthopedics, the trend is for subspecialization, with an additional year of fellowship training in such specialties as spine and hand surgery, sports medicine, and pediatrics.

Part VI features articles by a group of surgeons who subspecialize. They provide orthopedic treatment information for specific injuries, information that complements and augments that in Part III.

Neck and Back Surgery for Injuries in Outdoor Recreation

by David L. Coran, MD

Injuries of the back and neck are some of the most frequent reasons for doctor visits in the United States. Back and neck problems can occur in everyday life during work or recreational activities. They can be acute or chronic problems. Trauma, including falls and twisting accidents, can cause acute back and neck injuries, while chronic problems can recur without any precipitating event.

Understanding common back and neck problems is the first step in the prevention and treatment of these injuries.

People with chronic back and neck problems should be thoroughly evaluated and treated by a health care professional before participating in new outdoor recreational activities. Preexisting conditions of the spine may become aggravated during outdoor recreation, and symptoms of back and neck pain can return during participation in an activity.

When back and neck injuries occur for the first time during an outdoor recreational activity, it is important to have a basic knowledge of the different types of injuries to the spine so that appropriate treatment can be initiated.

The most common types of neck and back injuries are:

- Sprains and strains
- Disk herniations
- Fractures

Sprains and Strains

Sprains and strains are the most common types of injuries to the neck and back. A sprain or strain typically occurs with heavy lifting, twisting, and repetitive bending activities. Bending at the waist will commonly affect the lumbar (lower) back, while overhead lifting and repetitive bending of the neck are common causes of cervical (neck) sprains.

A sprain or strain injury usually involves a stretch or partial tear of a muscle, tendon, or ligament, which supports the lumbar or cervical spine.

Symptoms of sprains and strains of the neck and back include:

- Pain sensation, which is dull and aching
- Pain localized to the neck or lower back
- No radiation of pain or numbness into the arms or legs
- Severe pain with spasms of the muscles and difficulty walking may occur

The treatment of a sprain or strain is:

- Ice locally for the first 24 hours
- Nonsteroidal anti-inflammatory medications (such as aspirin or ibuprofen)
- Local heat after the first 24 hours
- Maintain activity—avoid bed rest
- No surgery

Disk Herniations

Disk herniations of the cervical or lumbar spine are less common than sprains and strains, but they can occur from the same types of activities. Repetitive bending, lifting, twisting, and overhead activity can lead to disk herniations. The continuous jarring of the spine, which occurs with running or bouncing, can also lead to disk injuries and herniations.

When a disk herniation occurs in the cervical or lumbar spine, the spinal cord or nerve roots can be affected. The disk structures are between the vertebrae (bones) of the spine and are in front of the nerve structures. When a disk herniates, it can apply pressure to the adjacent neural structures and lead to serious consequences.

Disk herniations in the cervical (neck) area can be the most serious due to the location of the spinal cord at this level. The spinal cord carries nerves to both the arms and legs, and an injury to the spinal cord can lead to paralysis. More typically, only a single nerve root is effected with a disk herniation, and symptoms are limited to the neck and arms.

Disk herniations in the lumbar spine (lower back) typically affect the nerve roots that supply the legs. The symptoms of numbness or weakness in either the arms or legs are signs of neurologic problems that suggest a more serious injury than a simple sprain or strain.

The symptoms of disk herniations in the neck or lower back include:

- Severe pain, which can radiate from the neck or lower back into the arms or legs.
- The pain can be severe, and walking or even sitting can be very difficult.
- Numbness or tingling in the arms or legs can occur frequently.
- Less commonly, weakness or even paralysis (inability to move the arms or legs) can occur.
- Changes in bowel or bladder function can rarely occur and represent medical emergencies.

The treatment of disk herniations initially is identical to that for sprains and strains unless there are associated "red flags":

- Difficulty emptying the bladder or controlling bowel movements, which could represent severe neurologic injury.
- Associated weakness of the arms or legs, which can progress to frank paralysis, also requires immediate medical attention.

Surgery is done when disk herniations cause one of the red flag warning signs above. The warning signs lead to further investigations by a physician, including plain x-rays and MRI studies of the injured area of the spine. The findings of large disk herniations pressing on the nerves or spinal cord would lead to a surgical procedure.

Surgery consists of removing the disk herniations, which then relieves the pressure on the neural structures. This is usually done by removing a small portion of bone from around the spine to gain access to the spinal canal where the disk herniation has occurred. Microsurgical and minimally invasive techniques have led to smaller incisions and faster recoveries for patients.

Even if there are no "red flags," medical attention should be sought if the pain persists for more than 7 days despite simple treatment measures.

Fractures

Fractures (broken bones) of the neck and back can occur with significant trauma, such as falls from heights, or high-speed activities, such as skiing. Whenever a fracture of the spine is suspected, immediate medical attention should be obtained to stabilize the injuries and prevent further damage to neurologic structures. A person with a suspected fracture should not be moved until experienced medical personnel are available to evaluate the situation and stabilize the spine appropriately.

Surgery is done when severe fractures occur. A patient with a fracture who is brought to medical attention requires extensive x-rays of the entire spine to look at the injured area as well as any associated injuries, which can occur in other regions of the spine when significant trauma occurs. Other medical problems can occur with spine fractures, including injuries to the internal organs of the chest and abdomen. These regions are also carefully evaluated with x-rays and CAT scans. A CAT scan provides a three-dimensional image of the internal structures and organs of the body.

When fractures are severe and become unstable, surgery is performed to fuse the unstable spine. Fusions often include the placement of metal screws and rods along the spine to support the fracture. If there is associated neurologic injury from the fracture and associated bone or disk fragments, these are removed at the time of surgery as well. Recovery is variable and depends on the severity of the injury.

Summary

Injuries of the neck and back are common with many outdoor recreational activities. They can be preexisting chronic problems, which become aggravated by outdoor activity. They can also occur for the first time during outdoor activities. The types of injuries range from minor sprains and strains to severe disk herniations or fractures. Fortunately, most injuries are minor and self-limiting.

Understanding how these injuries occur and how to recognize them when they occur can provide a basic background for treatment.

Being aware of the "red flags" of spinal injuries can prevent serious consequences from occurring.

Being involved in outdoor recreational activities is beneficial for a person's physical well-being. Appropriate preparation and care of the neck and back before and after activity should prevent the majority of injuries.

Dr. David L. Coran is an orthopedic spinal surgeon. He is a graduate of the University of Michigan Medical School and the Harvard Combined Orthopedic Program. He has also had fellowship training in the special fields of pediatrics and spinal surgery. His practice is devoted to the care of patients of all ages with spinal problems. When not practicing medicine, Dr. Coran enjoys golf, skiing, and running.

Treatment of Hand and Arm Injuries

by John A. Schneider, MD

Hand and arm injuries make up a large percentage of injuries from outdoor activities. These injuries can range from fractures to sprains and strains. Many of the injuries occur from repetitive use or trauma and can be avoided with proper conditioning and technique.

Common injuries of the hand and wrist include:

- Flexor tendon rupture (jersey finger)
- Extensor tendon rupture (mallet finger)
- Rupture of ulnar collateral ligament of thumb (skier's thumb)
- Scaphoid (navicular) fracture
- Median nerve impingement at the wrist (carpal tunnel syndrome)
- Ulnar neuritis at the wrist (biker's wrist)

Injuries involving the elbow include:

- Lateral epicondylitis (tennis elbow)
- Medial epicondyitis (baseball or golfer's elbow)
- Ulnar neuritis at the elbow (cubital tunnel syndrome)
- Distal biceps tendon rupture

Injuries involving the shoulder include:

- Acromioclavicular (AC) joint separation (shoulder separation)
- Glenohumeral joint dislocation (shoulder dislocation)
- Biceps tendon rupture
- Subacromial bursitis and rotator cuff tendinitis
- Rotator cuff tear

Flexor Tendon Rupture (Jersey Finger)

Injuries to the flexor tendons can result in inflammation or frank rupture of the tendons. The flexor tendon may be pulled off its bony attachment when excessive forces are applied to a contracting tendon. The most common cause of this type of injury is seen in football players when a finger catches the jersey of their opponent. This or similar injuries may also occur in rock climbing.

The treatment for minor injuries or inflammation of the tendons (tendinitis) is rest, anti-inflammatory medications, and stretching. This is followed by a strengthening program. Flexor tendon avulsions or tears usually always require operative treatment to repair the tendon. The surgery is followed by a very specific rehabilitation program that lasts approximately 12 weeks.

Extensor Tendon Rupture (Mallet Finger)

Ball sports are a common cause of extensor tendon injuries. They occur when a ball or other object strikes the extended fingertip. This strong force causes the thin ribbon-like extensor tendon to tear off its attachment at the end of the finger. This results in swelling and the inability to straighten the fingertip.

Most often these injuries are treated nonoperatively with an extended period of finger splinting. The joint toward the fingertip is held out straight, allowing the tendon to heal. Surgery is usually required only when a dislocation of the finger joint occurs along with the tendon injury.

Rupture of Ulnar Collateral Ligament of Thumb (Skier's Thumb)

Skiing and other activities that involve gripping an object may result in an injury to the thumb ulnar collateral ligament. This ligament is located at the ulnar (index finger side) of the large thumb joint. Excessive strain to the ligament, which can occur when falling with a ski pole in your hand, can cause a partial or complete tear. This renders the thumb unstable and painful with gripping or pinching.

Treatment of sprains (incomplete tear) of the ligament should involve ice, anti-inflammatory medication, and a period of immobilization. The length of immobilization depends on the severity of injury (4 to 8 weeks). Complete tears often require surgical repair of the ligament, followed by a course of immobilization.

Scaphoid (Navicular) Fracture

The scaphoid or navicular is a small bone located at the radial (thumb) side of the wrist. Falls onto the wrist that cause severe wrist extension (backwards bending) can cause fracture of this bone. On occasion this fracture can be confused with a severe wrist sprain. Indications of a fracture would be severe pain, bruising, or significant symptoms that persist beyond a few days. It is important to treat this fracture early, as it can be difficult to heal. Failure of the fractured scaphoid to heal often leads to severe arthritis of the wrist.

A scaphoid fracture that is not out of place can be treated with casting. Fractures that are displaced require surgical treatment to align the fracture. A screw is often used to hold the fracture together, allowing it to heal. Operative treatment of scaphoid fractures that are not out of place is becoming more common in patients with high physical demands, such as athletes, allowing for a quicker recovery with a shorter period of casting.

Median Nerve Impingement at the Wrist (Carpal Tunnel Syndrome)

Carpal tunnel syndrome is caused by impingement of the median nerve at the wrist. The median nerve runs down the center of the wrist and supplies sensation to the thumb, index, middle, and ring fingers, as well as controls the muscles about the thumb. Symptoms of carpal tunnel syndrome include pain at the wrist or thumb, weakness of grip, and numbness of the thumb, index, middle, or ring finger. These symptoms initially come and go. They become constant with increasing severity and duration of the impingement.

Repetitive activities involving the wrist and forearm and activities that require a fixed position of the wrist for long periods of time (particularly biking) can contribute to carpal tunnel syndrome. Usually multiple factors such as a small wrist size, arthritis, and general health conditions contribute to the development of carpal tunnel syndrome.

Initial treatment of carpal tunnel symptoms includes avoidance of aggravating activities, wrist and forearm stretching exercises, wearing gloves that pad the palm, and wrist splinting. If conservative measures fail to resolve the symptoms, surgical release of the carpal tunnel can be performed.

Ulnar Neuritis at the Wrist (Biker's Wrist)

The ulnar nerve, like the median nerve, can be impinged and irritated at the wrist. The ulnar nerve runs down the ulnar (small finger) side of the wrist. It supplies sensation to the small and ring fingers, as well as controls the small muscles of the hand. Signs of impingement of the ulnar nerve are numbness of the ring and small finger and loss of grip and pinch strength. Similar factors as those seen with carpal tunnel syndrome can contribute to ulnar neuritis. Direct pressure on the nerve for long periods, such as during biking, is a significant contributor to the problem. Trauma or a fall on the palm may also bring about symptoms.

Initial treatment consists of avoiding direct pressure on the ulnar nerve (small finger side of the hand) and wearing padded gloves. These measures usually improve the symptoms. Only rarely is surgical release of the ulnar nerve at the wrist required.

Lateral Epicondylitis (Tennis Elbow)

Lateral epicondylitis or tennis elbow occurs from repetitive injuries to the origin of the extensor muscles of the elbow. Symptoms consist of pain at the lateral (outside) portion of the elbow. This pain is increased with grasping objects, particularly with the elbow out straight and the palm facing downwards. Improper technique and tennis racquet grip size are common contributing factors to this problem.

Anti-inflammatory medications, icing the area, forearm stretching exercises, proper grip size, and avoidance of painful activities (lifting with the palm down and the elbow extended) are the initial steps in treating this problem. Formal therapy and cortisone injections can also be helpful. Surgical debridment and repair are reserved for those circumstances in which extensive conservative treatment has failed.

Medial Epicondyitis (Baseball or Golfer's Elbow)

Medial epicondylitis or baseball elbow is similar to lateral epicondylitis and occurs from repetitive injuries to the tendon origin at the medial (inside) aspect of the elbow. Pain is localized to the inside aspect of the elbow with throwing, swinging a golf club, or using a racquet.

Anti-inflammatory medications, icing the area, forearm stretching exercises, and avoidance of painful activities (lifting with the palm up and the elbow extended) are the initial steps in treating this problem. Formal therapy and cortisone injections can also be helpful, with surgical debridement and repair utilized for those circumstances when extensive conservative treatment has failed.

Ulnar Neuritis at the Elbow (Cubital Tunnel Syndrome)

Irritation or impingement of the ulnar nerve at the elbow (cubital tunnel syndrome) can occur from activities in which repetitive elbow flexion and extension are performed or when the elbow is held in a bent position for long periods of time. The ulnar nerve supplies sensation to the ring and small fingers, as well as supplies muscles of the forearm and hand. Symptoms of cubital tunnel syndrome include numbness or tingling of the small and ring fingers, weakness of grip and pinch, and pain at the medial aspect of the elbow.

Initial treatment of cubital tunnel syndrome involves forearm flexor and extensor stretching exercises, night splinting of the elbow in an extended (near straight) position, and avoidance of pressure on the nerve that runs at the medial aspect of the elbow. If symptoms persist despite these forms of conservative treatment, surgical release of the nerve may be performed.

Distal Biceps Tendon Rupture

The distal biceps tendon attaches to the radius (one of the forearm bones) at the elbow. The biceps muscle provides strength with flexion (bending) of the elbow as well as supination (twisting the palm upward, such as in using a screwdriver). Indications of rupture of this tendon are bruising about the elbow, deformity of the biceps muscle, and pain and weakness with elbow flexion and twisting of the forearm. Complete tears are often associated with the perception of a "pop."

Partial tears of the distal biceps tendon can be treated with a period of immobilization in a splint or cast, icing the area, and anti-inflammatory medications. Complete tears of the tendon are generally treated with surgical repair of the tendon back down to the bone. Newer techniques allow for early motion, limiting stiffness and providing for a faster recovery.

Acromioclavicular (AC) Joint Separation (Shoulder Separation)

Injuries to the acromioclavicular joint are common in activities such as hockey, football, and rugby. A blow to the outside aspect of the shoulder can cause pain, inflammation, and possibly separation of the AC joint. A separation occurs when the ligaments holding the clavicle to the shoulder bone (scapula) are disrupted. There are varying degrees of disruption that may occur related to the force of the injury.

The treatment of an AC joint separation that involves none or a mild amount of separation is immobilization in a sling, icing, and anti-inflammatory medications. As the ligaments heal, shoulder motion is initiated. Severely displaced shoulder separations require surgery to repair the ligaments and realign the AC joint.

Glenohumeral Joint Dislocation (Shoulder Dislocation)

The glenohumeral or ball-and-socket joint of the shoulder provides the shoulder with its large degree of motion. This joint consists of a shallow socket (glenoid) that the humeral head sits in. This joint can become dislocated if trauma causes disruption of the ligaments that hold the shoulder joint together. When this occurs, there is significant pain, deformity, and limited motion of the shoulder.

When a shoulder dislocation occurs, the initial treatment is reduction of the joint (placing the humeral head back on the glenoid), followed by a period of immobilization. Once the ligaments have had time to heal, motion and strengthening exercise of the shoulder are performed.

If the shoulder remains unstable or multiple dislocations occur, surgical repair of the ligaments and tightening of the glenohumeral joint are required.

Biceps Tendon Rupture

The biceps tendon has two attachments at its proximal, or shoulder, region. Rupture of the long head of the proximal biceps tendon can occur. This tendon enters the glenohumeral joint and is the thinner of the two proximal tendons. Signs of rupture of the long head of the biceps tendon include bruising, pain, and deformity of the proximal portion of the biceps muscle. Often the perception of a "pop" occurs at the time of injury.

Generally, no specific treatment other than comfort measures is performed for this injury. These include anti-inflammatory medications, icing the area, and possibly the use of a sling. Patients are usually pain free by 4 to 6 weeks. This injury produces minimal loss of function and weakness.

Subacromial Bursitis and Rotator Cuff Tendinitis

Subacromial bursitis occurs from performing repetitive overhead activities that cause pinching of the rotator cuff under the acromion (shoulder bone). When this occurs for an extended period of time, inflammation of the rotator cuff tendon (tendinitis) may occur. Symptoms include pain with motion of the shoulder, particularly with overhead reaching and reaching behind your back.

Initial treatment includes anti-inflammatory medications, shoulder range of motion exercises, physical therapy, and limitation of painful activities. This is followed by strengthening of the rotator cuff to help prevent recurrence of the problem. If these measures do not improve the symptoms, a cortisone injection into the subacromial space may be helpful. On rare occasions, surgical debridment is required.

Rotator Cuff Tear

Rotator cuff tears can occur from traumatic injuries, such as a fall on the shoulder, or they may occur over a long period of time due to impingement of the rotator cuff tendon. Symptoms of a rotator cuff tear are similar to that of rotator cuff tendinitis. They, however, are usually more severe, incompletely resolve with conservative treatment, and result in shoulder weakness.

Small, incomplete tears of the rotator cuff can heal with activity limitation, followed by shoulder range of motion exercises and strengthening. If the symptoms should persist or should there be a large tear of the rotator cuff, surgical repair is usually required. Repair of the torn rotator cuff tendon is performed back down to its previous site of attachment. After a period of immobilization, allowing the tendon to heal, range of motion exercises of the shoulder and rotator cuff strengthening are performed.

Summary

In summary, injuries to the upper extremity are common in outdoor activities. Many of these injuries can be prevented with appropriate conditioning, technique, and equipment. If you should develop pain or discomfort, the first step in treatment is avoidance of painful activities. Icing the affected area and anti-inflammatory medications can be helpful to aid in healing. Stretching and range of motion exercises should be performed once the symptoms resolve, followed by strengthening to get you back to your preinjury level of functioning. If symptoms persist or are severe, more formal medical treatment may be needed.

Dr. John A. Schneider is an orthopedic surgeon and specializes in the treatment of hand and upper extremity injuries. He is a graduate of Marquette University and attended medical school at the Medical College of Wisconsin. He performed his orthopedic surgery residency at the Creighton University/University of Nebraska program in orthopedic surgery and rehabilitation. In addition, he performed a hand and upper extremity fellowship at the Indiana Hand Center. Dr. Schneider participates in skiing, biking, running, and sailing.

Knee Pain in Recreational Biking and Running

by Harvey S. Kohn, MD

Knee pain is very common in recreational athletes. The knee is a central pivot area of the leg, and therefore it bears the brunt of force, which generates leg support activities. As we age, the normal process is accentuated by any degenerative changes that have occurred.

Knee Anatomy

The knee consists of external muscles that generate power, protect the internal structures of the knee, and connect the tibia to the femur bone. These muscles also incorporate the patella bone at the front of the knee, which helps protect the knee from injury and increases the efficiency of the muscles.

There are internal structures that guide and cushion movement. These consist of medial and lateral ligaments, anterior and posterior cruciate ligaments, menisci, and the articular cartilage surface (hyaline cartilage).

The muscles are the dynamic forces that can be trained for efficiency by systematic weight resistance activity and by sports-specific activities. That is, bikers have very large front thigh muscles and quadriceps muscles.

The internal structures, which connect the tibia to the femur, protect the knee from excessive side-to-side and front-to-back motion. These structures cannot be strengthened and are therefore known as static restraints. These guide motion and make precise bounding, jumping, running, and changing directions quickly possible. The joint surface of hyaline cartilage allows smooth motion to occur between the femur and tibia. Injury or naturally occurring wear can lead to pain and swelling of the knee.

The menisci are C-shaped fiber structures that cushion the knee during activities. The lateral meniscus lies on the outside of the knee. The medial meniscus lies on the inside of the knee between the femur and tibia bone. These can be injured by excessive stress, such as twisting as in a fall, or by cumulative wear over years of activity.

Specific knee conditions consist of:

- Muscle tendon inflammation, pulls, and tears
- Ligamentous strains and tears
- Tears to the menisci
- Injuries or excessive wear to the joint surfaces, including the patella

Muscle Tendon Injuries

The muscles act as a lever system to enable efficient motion to occur at the knee joint. Exceeding the strength of a muscle by a fall or sudden bend to the knee, as in stepping in a hole during running, a partial or complete tear can occur to the muscle or to the tendon. To avoid such injuries, a good strength and flexibility program can be instituted. Warm-up and stretching exercises before an activity are most helpful in preventing injuries. If a partial tear or pull occurs, ambulation is painful, running is most difficult, and medical care should be sought. A physician can assess muscle function and the degree of injury ascertained. An x-ray and MRI scan can assess the status of the bony structures and the muscle tendon structures. Protective weight bearing on crutches, a knee immobilizer, and a possible recommendation for surgery for repair in the case of a complete rupture or tear can be made. With modern orthopedic techniques of minimal excision and accelerated rehabilitation, the individual can be restored to recreational activities in a matter of months.

PATELLAR TENDINITIS

Patella tendinitis is a local inflammation of the tendon attachment of the patella to the tibia bone. It is caused by overuse, and results in pain during and after a workout and stiffness the next day. There is localized tenderness in this area and occasional swelling. Treatment consists of rest, ice, compression, and elevation (RICE), decreased running activities, including inclines, cross-training (biking and water activities), and physical therapy.

This diminishes the localized inflammation and strengthens the muscle unit attached to the tendon. A band similar to a tennis elbow band can be placed just below the patella to diminish stress when returning to running. Anti-inflammatory medication may be helpful in decreasing the inflammation. Once the localized pain diminishes, return back to activities can be graduated. Very occasionally, surgery to trim and repair the inflamed tendon is necessary to return to running after rehabilitation of 3 to 4 months.

IT BAND SYNDROME

The iliotibial (IT) band lies on the outer side of the knee joint. This is a large, flat band that can cause pain with excessive activities on uneven ground or occurs in the leg that is somewhat shorter than the opposite one. There is pain with palpation on the outer lateral knee (epicondyle), and a grating noise may occur with range of motion of the knee. These symptoms improve with diminished running. The treatment consists of diminishing the activity of workouts, cross-training, stretching for the excessively tight iliotibial bands by a physical therapist, and an orthotic or lift in the shoe for a shorter extremity. A steroid injection has proven to be very helpful, as well as selective use of anti-inflammatory medications.

The use of good supportive running shoes, especially in someone who is a pronator, is important, and use of orthotics by these people when returning to running may be quite helpful.

For more refractory conditions, surgery to release or lengthen this band may be necessary. Return to running after such an operation does not occur for a minimum of 3 to 4 months; however, cross-training can be carried out after 6 to 8 weeks.

Ligament Injuries

Ligaments can stretch or tear in recreational activities, as mentioned previously. A fall during running on uneven terrain is the most common injury by outer twisting of the knee. There are three grades of injury, grades I to III, which are mild, moderate, and severe. Mild sprains have less pain and swelling than severe ones. Treatment consists of the RICE principle with immobilization in a brace for 2 to 3 weeks. More severe injuries will generally heal on their own after a longer period of immobilization for 3 to 4 weeks and brace protection for another 3 to 4 weeks before return to activities. These injuries rarely, if ever, require surgery for repair of the ligament. Rehabilitation of the muscles following a period of immobilization is important in preventing recurrence and returning to biking and running activities.

ACL Injuries

Anterior cruciate ligament (ACL) injuries have received significant publicity in national news media over the last few years. They are recognized more commonly now, not overlooked and undertreated as they were 1 or 2 decades ago. They are unusual in runners and bikers except in crashes and falls.

Tears of the Menisci

The knee menisci are subject to stress through trauma, twisting, and by cumulative stresses by virtue of years of recreational activities. The former will be covered in another chapter. The latter is not an uncommon problem in the middle-age runner or bicyclist. Until 20 years ago, this condition wasn't well recognized except in obvious traumatic conditions, and runners and bikers were left to fend for themselves. Since then, with increasing recognition of this condition, diagnosis can be made and appropriate treatment rendered early on.

Symptoms consist of pain either on the inside or outside of the knee (depending on whether the lateral and medial meniscus is involved). With activities, locking, catching, or a piece of meniscus that is torn and caught in the joint occurs during activities, as well as possible swelling. A diagnosis made by physical exam with localized pain can be confirmed by an MRI examination.

Treatment consists of physical therapy to strengthen the muscle groups, bracing to protect the knee joint from buckling, anti-inflammatory medication to decrease pain and swelling, and diminishing activities (cross-training). If pain, swelling, locking, and catching persist, surgical arthroscopy to remove the torn piece of meniscus or to sew a tear of the meniscus back is very beneficial. The recovery period before returning to sports varies from 2 months for partial resection of the tissue to 4 months for repair.

Injuries and Wear to the Joint Surface

CHONDROMALACIA

Chondromalacia of the patella occurs commonly in biking, walking, and running activities, especially with hills and grade activities. Going down grades causes more problems than going up due to increasing strain on the kneecap by the quadriceps muscle. The condition is a cumulative one over time by virtue of running, biking, and walking. It is more common in individuals who are knock-kneed, in those with legs with increasing in-toeing of the foot (pronation), and in those with an imbalance of muscles around the knee (weaker inner thigh muscles than outer thigh muscles).

This leads to cartilage breakdown on the undersurface of the patella, and therefore pain in the front of the knee, stiffness before and after workouts, grating noise under the kneecap, and possibly swelling. The grading of this condition is from mild to moderately severe (grades I to IV).

Treatment consists of selective rest, cross-training, avoiding hills, wearing a patella sleeve or stabilizing brace, and physical therapy to balance the muscle forces across the knee. The RICE principle is also followed as mentioned above, and surgery to smooth the surface with an arthroscope as well as to rebalance the muscle forces may be necessary in chronic cases. The rehabilitation period to return to running and biking is at least 8 to 12 weeks following such a procedure.

OSTEOARTHRITIS

Osteoarthritis is excessive wear to the surface of the femur and tibia bone that can be due to the normal aging process or excessive stresses from years of activities. This can also be due to malalignment of the lower leg. Symptoms consist of pain and swelling with activity. There may be direct tenderness over the affected area on examination.

Treatment consists of cross-training, physical therapy to strengthen the muscles to relieve stress, anti-inflammatory medications, orthotics to help malalignment, supportive knee bracing, and good supportive running shoes. In addition, glucosamine and chondroitin sulfate are available over the counter and have been proven beneficial in mild to moderate conditions; for more refractory conditions, joint lubricant injections performed by a physician (hyaluronic acid such as Hyalgan) may be helpful symptomatically. Arthroscopic surgery to debride and smooth out the joint surfaces is not a long-term solution. Osteotomies, which cut the tibia and femur bone to correct malalignment, are used increasingly by orthopedic surgeons to relieve pain and slow the progression of changes to the joint surface. Total knee replacement for advanced conditions will relieve pain but will not return an individual to his or her accustomed running activities but should allow the individual to return to recreational walking and biking activities.

Summary

In conclusion, prevention of injuries by good strengthening and stretching programs and early recognition and treatment of these can greatly diminish frustration and lead to early return to specific activities.

Dr. Harvey S. Kohn is an avid recreational athlete, participating in running, tennis, golf, and weight lifting. He is a 1970 graduate of Albert Einstein College of Medicine and of New York Medical College orthopedic residency. He specializes in arthroscopy and sports medicine.

Twisting Injuries of the Knee in Outdoor Recreation

by Donald J. Zoltan, MD

Outdoor recreational activities are extremely popular worldwide, with millions of people participating in a wide variety of activities. Most people do not think of these activities as being high risk with regard to serious injuries; however, a significant amount of injuries do occur.

The knee is one of the most commonly injured joints in recreational activities. Twisting injuries of the knee can occur in both contact and noncontact settings.

The noncontact injuries are:

- Torn meniscus
- Anterior cruciate ligament (ACL) tear
- Quadriceps muscle tear
- Hamstring muscle tear
- Patella dislocation

The contact injuries are:

- Medial collateral ligament tear
- Posterior cruciate ligament tear
- Quadriceps contusion

Torn Meniscus

Knee injuries often involve meniscus tears (torn cartilage). The meniscus is a firm, rubbery, C-shaped tissue that helps cushion and stabilize the knee joint surface. Tears usually result from a twisting type of stress to the joint. The symptoms include painful locking and catching of the knee and a small to moderate amount of swelling. Swelling, if present, usually occurs the day after the injury.

Treatment for torn cartilage nearly always involves arthroscopic surgery. The arthroscope—a fiberoptic telescope approximately the size of a thin pencil—is used to repair or remove part of the torn meniscus. Whether the meniscus is repaired or removed depends on the extent or location of the tear.

Anterior Cruciate Ligament (ACL) Tear

Knee injuries that involve ligaments are usually the most serious. Ligaments are bands or sheets of fibrous tissue that connect bones to one another. One of the most serious knee ligament injuries involves the ACL. This ligament connects the tibia to the femur within the knee joint, and prevents excessive forward movement of the leg in relation to the thigh.

It is commonly thought that ACL tears can only occur from a direct contact blow to the knee; however, this is usually not the case. Tearing of the ligament is usually caused by a noncontact twisting injury. The twisting force that causes this ligament tear is usually much greater than the force that causes a meniscus tear. People will usually hear or feel a "pop" at the time of injury, and will notice a large amount of swelling an hour or two after the injury occurs.

Two treatment options are commonly recommended for ACL tears. One option involves a nonoperative approach. This requires an extensive physical therapy rehabilitation program to strengthen the quadriceps and hamstring muscles, and also involves obtaining a special stabilizing knee brace.

The other option of treatment involves ligament reconstruction surgery. This procedure is followed by an extensive physical therapy rehabilitation program. The type of treatment selected is determined by each person's desires and future recreational goals.

Quadriceps Muscle Tear

The quadriceps muscles are located in the front of the thigh and are responsible for straightening the knee. Tears, or muscles strains, usually occur from a sudden stretch of a contracted muscle. The result is pain, swelling, and weakness of the muscle.

Treatment of quadriceps muscle tears is nonsurgical. Initial treatment involves rest, ice, and elastic wrap compression.

After the acute inflammation subsides, stretching and strengthening exercise are initiated. Upon returning to vigorous outdoor activities, a Neoprene compression thigh sleeve is often beneficial.

Hamstring Muscle Tear

The hamstring muscles are located in the back of the thigh and are responsible for bending the knee. The cause, symptoms, and treatment are the same as that described for quadriceps muscle tears.

Patella Dislocation

The patella (kneecap) can pop out of joint with a significant twisting injury to the knee. When it dislocates toward the outside of the knee, most of the muscle and ligament attachments on the inside of the kneecap are torn. A large amount of knee swelling occurs almost immediately. A person may feel two "clunks" when this injury occurs, the first when the patella pops out of joint, and the second when it spontaneously slips back into place very soon after the dislocation.

The initial treatment of kneecap dislocation is nonsurgical. After the acute swelling subsides, a vigorous physical therapy rehabilitation program is initiated to strengthen the quadriceps muscles. Use of a patellar stabilizing brace upon return to recreational activities is also recommended.

Unfortunately, this nonoperative approach is sometimes unsuccessful. If recurrent dislocation should occur, surgical reconstruction to realign the patella is usually required.

Medial Collateral Ligament Tear

The medial collateral ligament, which extends from the thigh bone (femur) to the lower leg bone (tibia) on the inner side of the knee, can be injured by a direct blow to the outside of the knee. Pain and localized swelling are present on the inside of the knee.

Medial collateral ligament tears heal well without surgery. After a brief period of immobilization in a brace, a rehabilitation program is initiated emphasizing thigh muscle strengthening.

Posterior Cruciate Ligament Tear

The posterior cruciate ligament connects the femur to the tibia within the knee joint and prevents excessive backward movement of the leg in relation to the thigh. Unlike anterior cruciate ligament tears, posterior cruciate ligament tears are contact injuries. They occur from a direct impact to the front of the upper leg pushing the tibia in a backwards direction. In outdoor recreational activities, this occurs most commonly from a fall, when the ground makes contact with the front of the upper leg below the knee joint.

Initial treatment of posterior cruciate ligament tears is generally nonsurgical. Early immobilization followed by a vigorous physical therapy rehabilitation program stressing quadriceps strengthening is instituted. When full strength and flexibility are regained, return to full recreational activities is allowed, often with a special stabilizing brace. If persistent looseness and instability of the knee are present, surgical reconstruction of the posterior cruciate ligament can be considered.

Quadriceps Contusion

A direct impact injury to the front of the thigh can cause a quadriceps contusion, or deep thigh bruise, and results in pain, swelling, stiffness, and weakness of the muscle. This injury is often more serious than most people expect. While full recovery is anticipated, recovery time is often prolonged. Early muscle stretching is potentially harmful and should be delayed until later in the healing process.

Summary

Though not common in most outdoor recreational activities, serious twisting injuries of the knee can occur. These injuries can be classified as contact or non-contact. Treatment depends on the diagnosis, severity, and future recreational goals.

While some injuries are unavoidable, a certain percentage of injuries can be prevented. Proper conditioning, along with muscle stretching and strengthening programs, is an important preventative measure. In addition, proper equipment that is well adjusted to the individual is crucial. If an injury does occur, recognizing and treating it early in its course can help the individual return to activities as safely and quickly as possible.

Dr. Donald J. Zoltan is an orthopedic surgeon and enjoys golf, biking, and watching his children's baseball games. He is a graduate of Haverford College, the University of Ilinois Medical School, and completed his orthopedic residency at the University of Wisconsin. In addition, he attended the University of Florida for a sports medicine fellowship. His practice emphasizes arthroscopy, sports medicine, and joint replacements.

Pediatric Outdoor Recreation Injuries

by Brian E. Black, MD

In the past several years, running, hiking, and climbing have become increasingly popular among children and adolescents of both sexes. Consequently, outdoor injuries in children and adolescents have become more common.

The majority of pediatric running injuries are due to overuse and involve the apophyses. The apophyses are growth plates under tension from a musculotendinous insertion. Patellofemoral pain is another common problem among adolescent runners. Some of these injuries result from parents' and coaches' pressure to excel, as well as lack of knowledge about injury prevention.

It is safe for children to run. Children have been running in sports such as basketball and soccer for decades without too many problems. Guidelines for children's sports participation in running as a sport should be proper footwear, gradual progressive increase in distance and speed, and realistic and reasonable goals for children such as local competitions and shorter distances. Children should not run in marathons, for instance.

Some of the general treatment guidelines for children's running injuries are to modify the activity level, change to alternative exercises temporarily, and obtain better support for the legs and feet. Thermal treatments such as ice or heat and medications such as vitamins and nonsteroidal anti-inflammatory drugs (NSAIDs) or acetaminophen may be tried. In addition, a good surface and proper equipment help child runners return more readily to running as a sport. Healthful nutrition and appropriate adequate fluids are also necessary for these young athletes.

The following sections describe specific outdoor recreational injuries in adolescents and children and highlight their treatment.

Osgood-Schlatter Disease

Osgood-Schlatter should not be called a disease. It is a traction apophysitis of the tibial tubercle caused by repetitive traction trauma to the apophysis with a resulting tender prominence of the tibia tubercle. A lateral radiograph of the knee reveals this prominence, and a separate ossicle formation is often noted. Treatment consisting of temporary activity modification, icing after running, and optional use of a Chopat knee strap is usually adequate.

Severe recalcitrant cases can occasionally be treated in a knee immobilizer or cylinder cast. Very painful lesions persisting into adulthood sometimes require surgical removal of the ossicle through a patellar tendon-splitting approach. In the majority of cases, all pain is resolved by skeletal maturity.

Sinding-Larsen-Johansson Syndrome

Sinding-Larsen-Johansson syndrome is a traction apophysitis of the inferior patellar pole. Radiographically, slight separation and elongation of the inferior patellar pole are seen on the lateral view of the knee. Nonsurgical treatment is essentially the same as that of Osgood-Schlatter disease. All of these lesions adequately resolve by skeletal maturity without any need for surgery.

Adolescent Hip Pointer

Adolescent hip pointer is an avulsion injury of a musculotendinous origin from its pelvic apophysis. It may be either an acute or chronic injury. Treatment consists of rest, NSAIDs, and physical therapy modalities. These lesions heal at varying rates without the need for surgery. They are at times painful enough to require crutches temporarily.

Patellofemoral Pain Syndrome

Patellofemoral pain syndrome presents as generalized complaints of anterior knee pain without any history of trauma. This condition is particularly prevalent in female cross-country runners. Malalignment of the lower extremity is related to the development of patellofemoral pain syndrome. The malalignment findings typically are a constellation of foot pronation, external tibial torsion, genu valgum, and increased internal rotation at the hips. This malalignment causes the patella to track abnormally laterally.

Runners with patellofemoral pain syndrome typically complain of anterior knee pain, patellar instability, painful cracking from the patella, and the knee giving way. Their pain is increased by climbing stairs and hills.

Physical examination should evaluate patellar tracking with active knee flexion and extension. When the patella is passively pushed laterally, patients usually have apprehension from a sensation that the patella will subluxate or dislocate. The previously mentioned malalignment findings are usually present. The Q angle is greater than 20 degrees. Patellofemoral compression elicits pain.

Radiographic examination may reveal lateral tilting or subluxation on the patellar views. A lateral radiograph may demonstrate patella alta. The normal ratio of patellar length to patellar tendon length is no greater than 1:1.2. Increased patellar tendon length indicates patella alta, and a decrease indicates patella baja.

An appropriate physical therapy program should be faithfully pursued for at least 3 months before surgery is considered. Temporary use of a patellar stabilizing brace may allow patients to remain more asymptomatic during conservative treatment. Patients with pronated feet may find benefit from orthotics.

For the occasional patient who fails to respond to conservative management, surgical intervention is considered. Arthroscopic lateral release is usually the primary procedure of choice for a runner. The rehabilitation time is much shorter than with more extensive procedures. However, the surgeon and patient must be aware that lateral release has a high rate of failure (20 percent) and complications. Contraindications to lateral release are patella alta and excessive passive medial glide on examination.

For those runners for whom lateral release surgery fails or for whom it is contraindicated, proximal realignment procedures may be considered even for skeletally immature patients. Distal realignment procedures are contraindicated in skeletally immature patients but may be required for mature patients. Rehabilitation and a return to running are much more difficult for patients who undergo realignment procedures.

Adolescent and child runners also may be candidates for an additional procedure that is different from that in adults because of a child's open growth plates. Several of my patients with the malalignment syndrome and genu valgum have been successfully treated for their patellofemoral pain by distal medial femoral physeal stapling. Obviously, this technique cannot be useful in skeletally mature patients.

Sever's Apophysitis

Sever's apophysitis is a painful inflammatory condition of the apophysis of the calcaneal tuberosity. The pain may also extend into the plantar fascia or Achilles' tendon. Sever's apophysitis may be unilateral but most often occurs bilaterally. Heel pain occurs with weight-bearing activities. Tenderness on palpation of the calcaneal apophysis is noted on examination. An element of Achilles' tendon contracture is often observed. Radiographs are essentially nondiagnostic and are taken to rule out other pathologic conditions. Treatment consists of rest or activity modification, the use of viscoelastic heel cups or pedorthotics, NSAIDs, icing, Achilles' tendon stretching, and in severe recalcitrant cases, walking casts. Sever's apophysitis invariably resolves with closure of the calcaneal apophysis at skeletal maturity.

Stress Fractures

Stress fractures are rare in young runners and not uncommon in adolescents. Tibial or metatarsal sites are the most common. Runners often report a history of a recent increase in miles. Bone scan is the best early diagnostic tool because radiographs are often nondiagnostic. Rest is required until the symptoms resolve. This typically takes 4 to 6 weeks. Orthotics and proper shoes, both for better shock absorption, help prevent recurrence, particularly in runners with flat feet.

Summary

As outdoor recreation continues to grow in popularity for young patients, over-use injuries will continue to become more prevalent. In general, all of the conditions in this chapter are alleviated by modification of activity and other conservative measures. In many cases, as Frank Shorter has noted, "children are wonderfully self limiting." However, as running for sport becomes more important to young athletes and to their parents and coaches, orthopedists will continue to see increasing numbers of young enthusiasts with injuries and musculoskeletal problems.

Dr. Brian E. Black is the medical director of the Children's Orthopedic and Scoliosis Center and Spinal Performance Center in Milwaukee. He graduated from the University of Illinois College of Medicine and completed his residency in pediatric orthopedics at Johns Hopkins Hospital. He is board certified in orthopedic surgery by the American Board of Orthopedic Surgery. His special interests include children's orthopedics, scoliosis, injuries, cerebral palsy, birth defects, and hip, foot, and spine problems.

Foot Injuries in Outdoor Recreation

by Thomas A. Pietrocarlo, DPM

The foot is one of the most common areas of injury in avid walkers, climbers, hikers, and skiers. This is predictable when one considers the myriad of factors affecting the feet during these activities. These include shoe gear, structural variations in the feet, environmental factors, uneven terrain, cumulative mileage, and impact factors, to name a few.

The purpose of this chapter will be to cover some of the most common injuries. Each condition will be defined, the cause will be explained, and symptoms, treatment and prevention will be discussed.

Friction Blisters

A friction blister is a build-up of fluid or blood between the epidermis and dermal layer of skin caused by shearing forces applied to the skin.

Causes:

- Ill-fitting shoes (socks).
- Skin moisture.
- Pressure points on the foot.

Treatment:

- Drain using a sterile instrument (pin or knife cleaned with alcohol).
- Leave roof of blister intact.
- Apply antibiotic dressing.

Prevention:

- Reduce perspiration by applying topical antiperspirant.
- Identify areas of friction and pad them with moleskin.
- Check shoe fit.
- Wear socks that wick away moisture (polypropylene).
- Apply Vaseline to areas of friction.

Athlete's Foot

Athlete's foot infections are caused by a fungal infection of the skin. There are a variety of fungal organisms that can cause such infections.

Causes:

- Moisture, heat, and darkness, all of which occur in your shoes.

Symptoms:

- Itching, weeping, oozing, and skin macerations.
- Symptoms most commonly occur in the web spaces between the toes.
- Chronic cases may cause dry, scaly redness on the soles of the feet.

Treatment:

- Change socks frequently if wet, or use moisture-wicking socks (acrylic).
- Cleanse feet often.
- Apply topical antifungal creams until symptoms resolve and antifungal powders for preventative maintenance.

Prevention:

- Keep feet dry.
- Use an antifungal powder in shoes and socks.

Warts

A benign skin growth caused by a papilloma virus. A common skin condition in the foot.

Causes:

- Exposure to other individuals or surfaces that harbor the virus.
- Excessive perspiration of the feet can be a contributory factor.

Symptoms:

- Warts appear as painful bumps on the feet. They often bleed easily and are often confused as corns and calluses.
- They can occur on the soles of the feet (plantar warts) or toes.
- They are often painful when squeezed side to side.

Treatment:

- Initial treatment can be performed with over-the-counter products. Most of these include salicylic acid in various concentrations.
- Periodic paring down with a pumice stone.
- If unresponsive, seek professional help from a physician or podiatrist.

Prevention:

- Avoid going barefoot in communal environments (showers).
- Keep feet dry.

Black Toenails

A black toenail (subungual hematoma) is a build-up of blood beneath the nail plate. It may be acute, due to stubbing the toe or dropping a heavy object on the toe or chronic, due to repeated friction of the nail.

Causes:

- Acute or chronic injury to the nail.
- Improperly fitting shoes (too short, not enough room in the toe box).
- Repeated jamming of toes in boots, especially in downhill grades.

Symptoms:

- Acute pain in the toenail.
- Minimal pain but discoloration of the nail.
- Occasional bleeding and drainage from beneath the nail.

Treatment:

- If pain is acute, the hemorrhage beneath the toenail must be drained.
- In the field this can be done by heating a paperclip or sharp instrument and applying it to the nail plate until drainage occurs.
- A physician or clinic can decompress the nail with a high-speed drill or electrocautery.
- Chronic, nonpainful cases can be left alone. The nail will often grow out and eventually fall off, leaving a new nail beneath it.

Prevention:

- Careful fitting of shoes and socks.
- Avoidance of acute injuries to the toes.

Corns and Calluses

Corns and calluses are thickening of the skin caused by excessive localized pressure due to foot deformities or improperly fitting shoes.

Causes:

- Improperly fitting shoe.
- Foot deformities, such as bunions, hammertoes, and flat feet.

Symptoms:

- Painful thickening of skin usually over a bone prominence.
- Most common areas are the toes and balls of feet.

Treatment:

- Debride painful calluses with a pumice stone.
- Apply moisturizing creams daily.
- Pad areas of irritation with protective materials, including moleskin, felt and tape.
- Seek professional help from a podiatrist if symptoms persist.

Prevention:

- Check shoe fit to make certain there are no pressure points on the foot.
- Pad any bony prominences to avoid development.

Stress Fractures

A stress fracture is a partial or incomplete fracture of the bone due to repeated stress. The feet and ankles are the most common areas of involvement.

Causes:

- Repeated cyclic activities.
- May be predisposed to women with osteoporosis.
- Often occurs in nonconditioned athletes not accustomed to long walking or hiking.
- Certain athletes may be predisposed due to structural abnormalities in the feet.

Symptoms:

- Sudden onset of pain and swelling over the bone without a history of acute injury.
- Most common area in the foot is the metatarsal area (in-step area), although the heel and other areas are often injured.

Treatment:

- Immobilization and rest.
- Discontinue strenuous activities until symptoms are resolved.
- Seek medical evaluation and x-rays. Bone scan may be necessary if x-rays are negative.

Prevention:

- Slowly work into strenuous activities.
- Wear good supportive shock-absorbing shoe gear.
- If you suspect that you may have osteoporosis, seek medical advice from a physician.

Plantar Fasciitis

A chronic degenerative process causing inflammation of the plantar fascia (arch ligament) and often the development of a heel spur.

Causes:

- Foot type often predisposed to plantar fasciitis (i.e., flat or high arch feet).
- Improper shoes for a particular activity.
- Overuse.
- Obesity.
- Surface terrain.

Symptoms:

- Acute pain in the heel upon arising in the morning or after arising from a period of rest. The pain often extends into the arch area.
- Symptoms are often improved after being on your feet for a while but often return later in the day.

Treatment:

- Initially cutting back on athletic activities.
- Icing daily.
- Use of anti-inflammatory medications.
- Plantar fascia night splint.
- An arch support.
- Calf-stretching exercises.
- If symptoms fail to improve, consult with a podiatrist or physician for prescription of anti-inflammatory medications, physical therapy, and possibly prescription orthotics.

Prevention:

- Supportive shoe gear.
- Flexibility exercises for the calves.
- If you have flat feet, consider an arch support.

Haglund's Deformity

A Haglund's deformity is defined as an abnormal prominence of the posterior and superior aspect of the heel.

Causes:

- Often a congenital problem.
- More common in women.

Symptoms:

- Blister and callus formation over the posterior aspect of the heel.
- Repeated irritation and often swelling of the heel.
- A noticeable bony enlargement of the back of the heel.

Treatment:

- Calf stretching.
- Icing.
- Protection from irritation by padding the boot or heel with moleskin, felt, or foam.
- Surgery if symptoms become chronic.

Prevention:

- Careful boot fitting to avoid irritation.

Achilles Tendinitis

A traumatic or degenerative condition of the conjoined tendon of the calf muscle at or above its attachment to the heel.

Causes:

- Lack of Achilles tendon flexibility.
- Uphill walking, hiking, or climbing.
- Foot imbalances, such as flat or high arch feet, may be a predisposing problem.

Symptoms:

- Localized pain and swelling along the tendon.
- Pain when squeezing the tendon.

Treatment:

- Calf-stretching exercises before and after activities.
- Temporary heel lift in shoe or boot to relax the tendon.

- Icing.
- Anti-inflammatory medication.
- Arch supports if you have flat feet.
- Use of night splint to stretch the tendon.
- Avoidance of hills.
- Possibly physical therapy if symptoms fail to improve.
- Immobilization in a cast if symptoms fail to improve.

Prevention:

- Flexibility exercises for the calves.
- If you have a particular foot deformity, compensate by wearing an arch support.
- Slowly build up to hill climbing.

Neuroma

A neuroma represents an entrapment or compression of a nerve in the ball of the foot, usually between the third and fourth toes.

Causes:

- Tight-fitting shoes.
- Repeated flexion of the toes.
- Injury to the ball of the foot.

Symptoms:

- Numbness, burning, and pain to the adjacent third and fourth toes.
- Symptoms are exacerbated by tight-fitting shoes or repeated flexion of the toes.

Treatment:

- Shoes that are adequately wide.
- Stiffer toed shoes rather than those with flexible soles.
- Metatarsal padding.
- Possible steroid injection of the neuroma by a podiatrist or physician.
- Surgical removal if symptoms are unresponsive to conservative care.

Prevention:

- Shoes that are of adequate width.
- Stiffer soled shoes.

Ankle Sprains

An ankle sprain is a traumatic twisting injury usually involving the outer (lateral) ligaments of the ankle. The severity of the injury can vary from merely stretching the ligaments to a severe tear.

Cause:

- Acute inversion of the ankle usually due to uneven terrain.

Symptoms:

- Acute pain, swelling, and often discoloration over the outer aspect of the ankle.
- Often the outer ankle bone is very sore.
- A feeling of weakness in the ankle and inability to bear full weight.
- Discoloration will often occur on other areas of the foot as well.

Treatment:

- Ice, elevation, rest, compression.
- Splinting of the ankle.
- Anti-inflammatory medication.
- Examination by a podiatrist or physician to rule out a possible fracture or complete tear of the ligaments.
- Crutches if necessary.
- Physical therapy to reduce pain and symptoms and to rehabilitate the ankle.

Prevention:

- Supportive boot.
- Exercises for both strength and flexibility of the ankle.
- If you are prone to ankle sprains, a supportive brace may be helpful.

Bunion Deformity

A bunion is a complex deformity of the great toe joint resulting in a progressive dislocation. There is a progressive deformity of the foot, with the metatarsal bone protruding and the large toe moving in the opposite direction.

Causes:

- Hereditary factors.
- Women are more prone than men.
- Flat footedness.
- Tight-fitting shoes.

Symptoms:

- Persistent pain, irritation, redness, and blister formation over the prominent toe.
- Difficulty finding comfortable shoes.
- Often associated with other deformities, including hammertoes.

Treatment:

- Wider shoes to accommodate for the deformity.
- Softer upper on the shoes to avoid irritation.
- Arch supports when indicated (flat feet).
- Padding of the bunion to avoid irritation in shoe.
- Surgery if deformity is significant and unresponsive to conservative care.

Prevention:

- Careful shoe fit.
- Arch supports when indicated.

Hallux Rigidus

Hallux rigidus represents degenerative arthritis of the large toe joint. This is one of the most common areas of the foot to experience arthritis.

Causes:

- Major trauma to the joint.
- Repeated minor injuries to the joint.
- Hereditary variation in the alignment of the joint.

Symptoms:

- Pain and stiffness in the large toe.
- Inability to push off with the large toe.
- Enlargement of the great toe joint with resultant shoe irritation.

Treatment:

- Stiff soled shoes with a deep toe box to accommodate for the deformity.
- Icing.
- Anti-inflammatory medications.
- Orthotics.
- Surgery to correct the deformity. Various surgical procedures can be performed, ranging from cleaning up the joint, joint fusion, to joint replacement.

Prevention:

- Avoiding of injury with stiff-toed shoes.

Hammertoes

A hammertoe is a deformity of the lesser toes characterized by contraction of the toe.

Causes:

- Hereditary.
- Poor shoes.
- Foot imbalances (high and low arch).
- Often associated with bunion deformity.

Symptoms:

- Painful irritation of the top of the toes.
- Corn formation.
- Pain on balls of feet.

Treatment:

- Deep toe box shoes.
- Padding to avoid irritation.
- Surgery if all measures fail.

Prevention:

- Shoes with deep toe box.
- Arch support if indicated.

Summary

This chapter should serve to familiarize you with some of the more common foot and ankle injuries that can occur in outdoor recreational activities. There are many other conditions that can occur that are not included. If there are any doubts as to the type of injury or failure to respond to treatment, you should consult a health care professional.

Dr. Thomas A. Pietrocarlo is a podiatrist who has been practicing in the Milwaukee area for the past 25 years. He is a graduate of the Ohio College of Podiatric Medicine. His special interests are in the area of foot surgery and sports medicine. He has authored numerous articles on foot and ankle problems in athletes. His professional affiliations include clinical instructor, Medical College of Wisconsin; diplomate, American Board of Podiatric Surgery; fellow, American College of Foot and Ankle Surgeons; and member, American College of Sports Medicine.

AC (acromioclavicular) joint separation, 61–64, 270
  condition statement, 61–62
  rehabilitation exercises, 194–96
  treatment plan, 63–64
Achilles tendinitis, 161–63, 291–92
  condition statement, 161–62
  rehabilitation exercises, 182–84, 210–13
  treatment plan, 162–63
Achilles tendon, torn, 164–66
  condition statement, 164–65
  rehabilitation exercises, 210–13
  treatment plan, 165–66
ACL (anterior cruciate ligament) tear, 123–26, 275, 278–79
  condition statement, 123–24
  rehabilitation exercises, 208–9
  treatment plan, 125–26
acromioclavicular (AC) joint separation, 61–64, 270
  condition statement, 61–62
  rehabilitation exercises, 194–96
  treatment plan, 63–64
activity alternatives, in treatment plan, 23–24
activity levels, in treatment plan, 22–23
acute traumatic injuries, 16
adductor muscle tear, 103–6
  condition statement, 103–4
  rehabilitation exercises, 182–84
  treatment plan, 104–6
adolescent hip pointer, 283
allergic causes of pain and injury, 18
ankle injuries. *See also* foot injuries
  achilles tendinitis, 161–63, 291–92
  lateral ligament sprain, 167–69, 293
  rehabilitation exercises, 182–84, 210–13
  Sever's apophysitis, 284
  sprain, 293
  stress fracture, 284, 289–90
  torn Achilles tendon, 164–66
ankle sprain, 293
anterior cruciate ligament tear, 123–26, 275, 278–79

condition statement, 123–24
  rehabilitation exercises, 208–9
  treatment plan, 125–26
anterior dislocation, 65–68, 270
  condition statement, 65–66
  rehabilitation exercises, 197–99
  treatment plan, 67–68
anti-inflammatory medications, 31–32
antioxidants, 236–37
arm and hand injury treatment, 266–72.
  See also elbow injuries; shoulder injuries; wrist injuries
arthrogram, 19
arthroscopy, 20
athlete's foot, 286–87

back injuries
  herniated or slipped disk, 54–57, 263–64
  muscle tear, 58–60
  rehabilitation exercises, 181–86
  sprain and strain, 262–63
  surgery for, 262–65
back strengthening program, 184–86
baseball elbow, 82–84, 269
  condition statement, 82–83
  rehabilitation exercises, 200–204
  treatment plan, 83–84
baseball finger, 97–99, 267
  condition statement, 97–98
  rehabilitation exercises, 200–201
  treatment plan, 98–99
biceps tendon rupture, 73–75, 270–71
  condition statement, 73–74
  rehabilitation exercises, 187–89, 194–96
  treatment plan, 74–75
biceps tendon rupture, distal, 269–70
bicycle paths, 39
bicycles, 34
biker's wrist, 94–96, 268
  condition statement, 94–95
  rehabilitation exercises, 200–204
  treatment plan, 95–96
biking, knee pain in, 273–77

black toenails, 288
blacktop surfaces, 39
blisters, friction, 286
bone scan, 19
braces, 27–28
breakfast, 216
bunion deformity, 293–94
bursitis, subacromial, 76–78
    condition statement, 76–77
    rehabilitation exercises, 187–93
    treatment plan, 77–78
bursitis, trochanteric, 111–13
    condition statement, 111–12
    rehabilitation exercises, 182–84
    treatment plan, 112–13

calf injury, 157–60, 210–13
calluses and corns, 288–89
calories, 217, 218–19
carbohydrates, 219–25
    requirements, 223–25
    types, 220–21
carpal tunnel, 88–90, 268
    condition statement, 88–89
    rehabilitation exercises, 200–204
    treatment plan, 89–90
CAT scan, 20
causes of injuries, 14–15
chest injury, 51–53, 181–84
children's injuries, 282–85
chiropractors, 7
cholesterol, 37
chondromalacia patella, 127–30, 276
    condition statement, 127–28
    rehabilitation exercises, 204–6
    treatment plan, 129–30
chronic overuse injuries, 16
climbing injury prevention, 253–59
    clothing, 255–56
    equipment, 256–58
    hiking etiquette, 258–59
    preparing for hike, 253–58
    survival tips, 258
coaches, as source of information, 8
computerized axial tomography scan, 20
concrete surfaces, 39
condition summary, 6-point, 17–21. See also
        specific injuries
congenital causes of pain and injury, 18
contusion, quadriceps, 280
corns and calluses, 288–89
COX inhibitors, 32
cramps, muscle, 235

cross-country ski machines, 33–34
cubital tunnel syndrome, 269

dairy foods, 227
degenerative causes of pain and injury, 18
delayed pain, 23
diet. See nutrition and diet
disk herniations (back), 54–57, 263–64
    condition statement, 54–55
    rehabilitation exercises, 182–86
    treatment plan, 56–57
disk herniations (neck), 47–50, 263–64
    condition statement, 47–48
    rehabilitation exercises, 181–82
    treatment plan, 48–50
dislocation, anterior, 65–68, 270
    condition statement, 65–66
    rehabilitation exercises, 197–99
    treatment plan, 67–68
dislocation, kneecap, 141–45, 279–80
    condition statement, 141–42
    rehabilitation exercises, 204–9
    treatment plan, 143–44
distal biceps tendon rupture, 269–70. See
        also biceps tendon rupture

eating. See nutrition and diet
eggs, 227
EKG (electrocardiogram), 20
elbow injuries
    lateral epicondylitis (tennis elbow),
        79–81, 268–69
    medial epicondylitis (baseball elbow),
        82–84, 269
    rehabilitation exercises, 200–204
    ulnar nerve entrapment, 85–87
    ulnar neuritis, 269
elliptical trainers, 34
EMG (electromyogram), 20
endurance, 24–25
equipment, in treatment plan, 32–36
exercise. See also specific injuries
    reasons for, 4
    rehabilitation programs, 24–27
    reward/risk ratio, 2–4
    using equipment, 26–27
extensor tendon tear, 97–99, 267
    condition statement, 97–98
    rehabilitation exercises, 200–201
    treatment plan, 98–99

fat, 228–33
    requirements, 228–29

types, 229–31, 236–37
femur, stress fracture of neck of, 107–10
  condition statement, 107–8
  rehabilitation exercises, 182–84
  treatment plan, 109–10
fibula or tibia stress fracture, 154–56
  condition statement, 154–55
  rehabilitation exercises, 182–84, 210–13
  treatment plan, 155–56
finger injuries
  extensor tendon tear (baseball finger),
    97–99, 267
  flexor tendon rupture, 266–67
  rehabilitation exercises, 200–201
  ruptured ulnar collateral ligament (skier's
    thumb), 100–102, 267
flexibility, 24–25
flexor tendon rupture, 266–67
fluids, 37–38, 217, 233–35
foot injuries, 286–96. See also ankle injuries
  athlete's foot, 286–87
  black toenails, 288
  bunion deformity, 293–94
  corns and calluses, 288–89
  friction blisters, 286
  Haglund's deformity, 291
  hallux rigidus, 294–95
  hammertoes, 295
  metatarsal stress fracture, 170–72
  Morton's neuroma, 173–75
  neuroma, 292–93
  plantar fasciitis, 176–78, 290
  rehabilitation exercises, 182–84, 210–13
  stress fracture, 284, 289–90
  warts, 287–88
fractures
  back, 264
  femur neck, 107–10, 182–84
  foot, 284, 289–90
  metatarsal, 170–72, 182–84, 210–13
  neck, 264
  scaphoid bone, 91–93, 200–204, 267
  tibia or fibula, 154–56, 182–84, 210–13
  vertebra and rib, 51–53, 181–84
friction blisters, 286
friends, as source of information, 8

gastrocnemius muscle rupture, 157–60
  condition statement, 157–58
  rehabilitation exercises, 210–13
  treatment plan, 158–60
glenohumeral joint dislocation, 65–68, 270
glycemic index, 222–23

golfer's elbow, 82–84, 269
  condition statement, 82–83
  rehabilitation exercises, 200–204
  treatment plan, 83–84

Haglund's deformity, 291
hallux rigidus, 294–95
hammertoes, 295
hamstring muscle tear, 120–22, 279
  condition statement, 120–21
  rehabilitation exercises, 182–84, 208–9
  treatment plan, 121–22
hand and arm injury treatment, 266–72. See
    also elbow injuries; shoulder injuries;
    wrist injuries
heat, in treatment of sports injuries, 30
heel pain, 176–78, 290
  condition statement, 176–77
  rehabilitation exercises, 182–84, 210–13
  treatment plan, 177–78
herniated disk (neck), 47–50, 263–64
  condition statement, 47–48
  rehabilitation exercises, 181–82
  treatment plan, 48–50
herniated or slipped disk (back), 54–57,
    263–64
  condition statement, 54–55
  rehabilitation exercises, 182–86
  treatment plan, 56–57
heterotopic bone formation, 114–16
  condition statement, 114–15
  rehabilitation exercises, 204–9
  treatment plan, 115–16
hiking. See also climbing injury prevention;
    pole use
  etiquette, 258–59
  with poles, 249–50
  preparing for, 253–58
hiking poles, 240–41. See also pole use
hip injuries
  adductor muscle tear, 103–6
  adolescent hip pointer, 283
  rehabilitation exercises, 182–84
  stress fracture of neck of femur, 107–10
  trochanteric bursitis, 111–13

ice, in treatment of sports injuries, 29–30
iliotibial band syndrome, 131–33, 274–75
  condition statement, 131–32
  rehabilitation exercises, 204–9
  treatment plan, 132–33
indoor paths, 39
infection, as cause of pain and injury, 18

injury causes, 14–15
injury form, 10
injury prevention, 215–59
    in hiking, rock climbing and
        mountaineering, 253–59
    with nutrition and diet, 216–38
    with pole use, 239–52
injury types, 15–16
instability, 5–6
isokinetic machines, 26–27
isometric exercises, 26
isotonic exercises, 26
IT (iliotibial band) syndrome, 131–33, 274–75
    condition statement, 131–32
    rehabilitation exercises, 204–9
    treatment plan, 132–33

jersey finger, 266–67
jumper's knee, 145–47, 274
    condition statement, 145–46
    rehabilitation exercises, 204–9
    treatment plan, 146–47

Kenalog, 32
knee anatomy, 273
knee braces, 27–28
kneecap dislocation, 141–45, 279–80
    condition statement, 141–42
    rehabilitation exercises, 204–9
    treatment plan, 143–44
knee injuries
    anterior cruciate ligament tear, 123–26,
        275, 278–79
    chondromalacia patella, 127–30, 276
    iliotibial band syndrome, 131–33, 274–75
    to joint surface, 276–77
    kneecap dislocation, 141–45, 279–80
    ligament injuries, 275
    medial collateral ligament tear, 280
    muscle tendon injuries, 274–75
    Osgood-Schlatter disease, 134–36, 282
    osteoarthritis, 137–40, 276–77
    patellar tendinitis (jumper's knee),
        145–47, 274
    patellofemoral pain syndrome, 283–84
    posterior cruciate ligament tear, 280
    rehabilitation exercises, 182–84, 204–9
    Sinding-Larsen-Johansson syndrome, 283
    torn meniscus, 148–50, 275–76, 278
    twisting injuries, 278–81
knee pain in biking and running, 273–77

lateral epicondylitis, 79–81, 268–69

condition statement, 79–80
    rehabilitation exercises, 200–204
    treatment plan, 80–81
lateral ligament sprain, 167–69, 293
    condition statement, 167–68
    rehabilitation exercises, 210–13
    treatment plan, 168–69
listening to your body, 1–11
    methods, 4–6
    outside support, 6–11
    reasons for, 1–4
localized pain, 22–23
lower extremity stretching program,
    182–84

magnetic resonance imaging (MRI), 20
mallet finger, 97–99, 267
    condition statement, 97–98
    rehabilitation exercises, 200–201
    treatment plan, 98–99
meat, red, 227
mechanical causes of pain and injury, 18
medial collateral ligament tear, 280
medial epicondylitis, 82–84, 269
    condition statement, 82–83
    rehabilitation exercises, 200–204
    treatment plan, 83–84
median impingement at the wrist,
    88–90, 268
    condition statement, 88–89
    rehabilitation exercises, 200–204
    treatment plan, 89–90
medical doctors, 7, 9–11
medications, 31–32
meniscus, torn, 148–50, 275–76, 278
    condition statement, 148–49
    rehabilitation exercises, 182–84, 206–7
    treatment plan, 149–50
meniscus program, 206–7
metabolic causes of pain and injury, 18
metabolic differences, 218
metatarsal stress fracture, 170–72
    condition statement, 170–71
    rehabilitation exercises, 182–84, 210–13
    treatment plan, 171–72
monounsaturated fatty acids, 231
Morton's neuroma, 173–75
    condition statement, 173–74
    rehabilitation exercises, 182–84, 210–13
    treatment plan, 174–75
MRI (magnetic resonance imaging), 20
muscle cramps, 235
muscle soreness, 235–36

muscle tear, back, 58–60
    condition statement, 58–59
    rehabilitation exercises, 181–86
    treatment plan, 59–60
myelogram, 19
myositis ossificans, 114–16
    condition statement, 114–15
    rehabilitation exercises, 204–9
    treatment plan, 115–16

navicular bone fracture, 91–93, 267
    condition statement, 91–92
    rehabilitation exercises, 200–204
    treatment plan, 92–93
neck injuries
    herniated disk, 47–50, 263–64
    rehabilitation exercises, 181–82
    sprain and strain, 262–63
    surgery for, 262–65
neck of femur stress fracture, 107–10
    condition statement, 107–8
    rehabilitation exercises, 182–84
    treatment plan, 109–10
neuroma, 292–93
noise, in joints, 5
Nordic/fitness poles, 241–43. *See also*
        pole use
nurses, 7
nutrition and diet, 216–38
    antioxidants, 236–37
    carbohydrates, 219–25
    fat, 228–33, 236–37
    general tips, 216–19
    goals, 218
    injury prevention, 235–36
    protein, 225–27
    in treatment plan, 36–37
    water, 37–38, 217, 233–35

omega-3 fatty acids, 229–31, 236–37
omega-6 fatty acids, 229–31
orthopedic surgeons, 7
Osgood-Schlatter disease, 134–36, 282
    condition statement, 134–35
    rehabilitation exercises, 182–84, 204–9
    treatment plan, 135–36
osteoarthritis, 137–40, 276–77
    condition statement, 137–38
    rehabilitation exercises, 182–84, 204–9
    treatment plan, 139–40
osteopaths, 7
over-the-counter medications, 32
overuse injuries, chronic, 16

pain
    causes, 18
    knee pain in biking and running, 273–77
    as symptom, 4–5
    types, 22–23
pain, heel, 176–78, 290
    condition statement, 176–77
    rehabilitation exercises, 182–84, 210–13
    treatment plan, 177–78
parents, as source of information, 8
patella dislocation, 141–45, 279–80
    condition statement, 141–42
    rehabilitation exercises, 204–9
    treatment plan, 143–44
patellar program, 204–6
patellar tendinitis, 145–47, 274
    condition statement, 145–46
    rehabilitation exercises, 204–9
    treatment plan, 146–47
patellofemoral pain syndrome, 283–84
pediatric injuries, 282–85
physical therapists, 7
physicians, 7, 9–11
plantar fasciitis, 176–78, 290
    condition statement, 176–77
    rehabilitation exercises, 182–84, 210–13
    treatment plan, 177–78
podiatrists, 7
pole use, 239–52
    absence of pain, 251–52
    benefits of walking with poles, 244–45
    for disease and injury prevention and
        rehabilitation, 250–51
    evolution of fitness poles, 239–40
    fitness walking with poles, 243–45
    hiking and trekking with poles, 249–50
    methods, 245–49
    pole types, 240–43
    sizing poles, 243
polyunsaturated fatty acids, 229–31, 236–37
posterior cruciate ligament tear, 280
protein, 225–27
psychogenic causes of pain and injury, 18

quadriceps contusion, 280
quadriceps muscle tear, 117–19, 279
    condition statement, 117–18
    rehabilitation exercises, 204–9
    treatment plan, 118–19

radionuclide, 19
rehabilitation exercise programs. *See also*
        specific injuries

ankle, 210–13
anterior cruciate ligament, 208–9
back strengthening, 184–86
lateral epicondylitis (advanced), 202–4
lateral epicondylitis (beginning), 200–201
lower extremity stretching, 182–84
meniscus, 206–7
overview, 179–80
patellar, 204–6
rotator cuff, 190–93
shoulder acromioclavicular, 194–96
shoulder (beginning), 187–89
shoulder dislocation, 197–99
in treatment plan, 24–27
upper extremity stretching, 181–82
rib and vertebra fracture, 51–53
RICE (rest, ice, compression, elevation),
   29–30
roentgenograms, 19
rotator cuff tendinitis and tear, 69–72, 271
condition statement, 69–70
rehabilitation exercises, 187–93
treatment plan, 71–72
rowing machines, 34
running, knee pain in, 273–77
rupture, biceps tendon, 73–75, 270–71
condition statement, 73–74
rehabilitation exercises, 187–89, 194–96
treatment plan, 74–75
rupture, flexor tendon, 266–67
rupture, gastrocnemius muscle, 157–60
condition statement, 157–58
rehabilitation exercises, 210–13
treatment plan, 158–60
rupture, ulnar collateral ligament,
   100–102, 267
condition statement, 100–101
rehabilitation exercises, 200–201
treatment plan, 101–2

saturated fatty acids, 231–32
scaphoid bone fracture (navicular bone),
   91–93, 267
condition statement, 91–92
rehabilitation exercises, 200–204
treatment plan, 92–93
Sever's apophysis, 284
shin injuries
rehabilitation exercises, 182–84, 210–13
shin splints, 151–53
tibia or fibula stress fracture, 154–56
shin splints, 151–53
condition statement, 151–52

rehabilitation exercises, 182–84, 210–13
treatment plan, 152–53
shoes, 35–36
shoulder dislocation, 65–68, 270
condition statement, 65–66
rehabilitation exercises, 197–99
treatment plan, 67–68
shoulder injuries
acromioclavicular joint separation,
   61–64, 270
anterior dislocation, 65–68, 270
biceps tendon rupture, 73–75, 270–71
rehabilitation exercises, 187–96
rotator cuff tendinitis and tear,
   69–72, 271
subacromial bursitis, 76–78
Sinding-Larsen-Johansson syndrome, 283
skier's thumb, 100–102, 267
condition statement, 100–101
rehabilitation exercises, 200–201
treatment plan, 101–2
slipped disk (back), 54–57, 263–64
condition statement, 54–55
rehabilitation exercises, 182–86
treatment plan, 56–57
soreness, muscle, 235–36
speed, 15, 24–25
sprain, ankle, 293
sprain, lateral ligament, 167–69, 293
condition statement, 167–68
rehabilitation exercises, 210–13
treatment plan, 168–69
sprain, neck and back, 262–63
stiffness, 5
Stop, Yield, Go concept, 17
and activity levels, 22
and alternative activities, 23
and equipment, 33
and fluids, 37
and medication, 31
and nutrition, 36
and rehabilitation exercises, 25
and support, 28
and surfaces, 387
and thermal treatment, 28
strain, neck and back, 262–63
strength, 24–25
strengthening program, back, 184–86
stress fracture, foot, 284, 289–90
stress fracture, metatarsal, 170–72
condition statement, 170–71
rehabilitation exercises, 182–84, 210–13
treatment plan, 171–72

stress fracture, neck of femur, 107–10
  condition statement, 107–8
  rehabilitation exercises, 182–84
  treatment plan, 109–10
stress fracture, tibia or fibula, 154–56
  condition statement, 154–55
  rehabilitation exercises, 182–84, 210–13
  treatment plan, 155–56
stretching, 25–26
  lower extremity, 182–84
  upper extremity, 181–82
subacromial bursitis, 76–78
  condition statement, 76–77
  rehabilitation exercises, 187–93
  treatment plan, 77–78, 271
support, in treatment plan, 27–28
surfaces, in treatment plan, 38–39
surgery, neck and back, 262–65
swelling, 5

teachers, as source of information, 8
tendinitis, Achilles, 161–63, 291–92
  condition statement, 161–62
  rehabilitation exercises, 182–84, 210–13
  treatment plan, 162–63
tendinitis, patellar, 145–47, 274
  condition statement, 145–46
  rehabilitation exercises, 204–9
  treatment plan, 146–47
tendinitis, rotator cuff, 69–72, 271
  condition statement, 69–70
  rehabilitation exercises, 187–93
  treatment plan, 71–72
tennis elbow, 79–81, 268–69
  condition statement, 79–80
  rehabilitation exercises, 200–204
  treatment plan, 80–81
testing procedures, 19–21
thermal treatment, 28–30
thermogram, 19
thigh injuries
  adductor muscle tear, 103–6
  hamstring muscle tear, 120–22, 279
  myositis ossificans, 114–16
  quadriceps contusion, 280
  quadriceps muscle tear, 117–19, 279
  rehabilitation exercises, 182–84, 204–9
tibia or fibula stress fracture, 154–56
  condition statement, 154–55
  rehabilitation exercises, 182–84, 210–13
  treatment plan, 155–56
toenails, black, 288

trainers, as source of information, 7–8
trans fatty acids, 232–33
traumatic causes of pain and injury, 18
traumatic injuries, acute, 16
treadmills, 33
treatment plan, 10-point, 21–39. *See also*
  specific injuries
trekking with poles, 240, 249–50. *See also*
  pole use
trochanteric bursitis, 111–13
  condition statement, 111–12
  rehabilitation exercises, 182–84
  treatment plan, 112–13
tumors, as cause of pain and injury, 18
twisting injuries, 15, 278–81
types of injuries, 15–16

ulnar collateral ligament rupture,
  100–102, 267
  condition statement, 100–101
  rehabilitation exercises, 200–201
  treatment plan, 101–2
ulnar nerve entrapment, 85–87
  condition statement, 85–86
  rehabilitation exercises, 200–204
  treatment plan, 86–87
ulnar neuritis, elbow, 269
ulnar neuritis, wrist, 94–96, 268
  condition statement, 94–95
  rehabilitation exercises, 200–204
  treatment plan, 95–96
upper extremity stretching program, 181–82

vague pain, 22
vascular causes of pain and injury, 18
vertebra and rib fracture, 51–53
  condition statement, 51–52
  rehabilitation exercises, 181–84
  treatment plan, 52–53

warts, 287–88
water, drinking, 37–38, 217, 233–35
weight lifting equipment, 34–35
wood surfaces, 39
wrist injuries
  carpal tunnel, 88–90, 268
  rehabilitation exercises, 200–204
  scaphoid bone fracture, 91–93, 267
ulnar neuritis (biker's wrist), 94–96, 268

x-rays, 19

About the Author

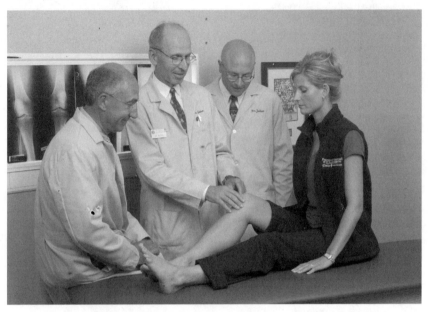

Dr. Gary Guten (center) teams up with Drs. Donald Zoltan (left) and Thomas Pietrocarlo (right) to examine the knee of physical therapist Andrea Vanderveldt.

Orthopedic surgeon Gary N. Guten, MD, is an expert in the treatment of sports injuries. As founder of the Sports Medicine and Orthopedic Center in Milwaukee, senior medical advisor for the Sports Medicine and Performance Center at St. Francis Hospital in Milwaukee, and former team physician for the Milwaukee Brewers professional baseball team, he treats hundreds of athletes and outdoor recreational enthusiasts every year. A marathon runner, bicyclist, hiker, and golfer, Guten lives in Milwaukee.